P9-CBG-531

David F. Fardon, M.D.

FREE YOURSELF FROM BACK PAIN

Prentice-Hall, Inc., Englewood Cliffs, N.J. 07632

Library of Congress Cataloging in Publication Data

Fardon, David F.
  Free yourself from back pain.

  1. Backache—Treatment.   2. Backache—Prevention.
3. Exercise therapy. I. Title.
RD768.F37   1984   617'.56   84-4731
ISBN 0-13-330655-0
ISBN 0-13-330648-8 (pbk.)

© 1984 by Prentice-Hall, Inc., Englewood Cliffs, New Jersey 07632.
All rights reserved. No part of this book may be reproduced in any form
or by any means without permission in writing from the publisher.
Printed in the United States of America.

2   3   4   5   6   7   8   9   10

ISBN 0-13-330655-0

ISBN 0-13-330648-8 {PBK.}

Editorial/production supervision by Peter Jordan
Cover design by Hal Siegel
Manufacturing buyer: Pat Mahoney

This book is available at a special discount when ordered in
bulk quantities. Contact Prentice-Hall, Inc., General
Publishing Division, Special Sales, Englewood Cliffs, N.J. 07632.

Prentice-Hall International, Inc., *London*
Prentice-Hall of Australia Pty. Limited, *Sydney*
Prentice-Hall Canada Inc., *Toronto*
Prentice-Hall of India Private Limited, *New Delhi*
Prentice-Hall of Japan, Inc., *Tokyo*
Prentice-Hall of Southeast Asia Pte. Ltd., *Singapore*
Whitehall Books Limited, *Wellington, New Zealand*
Editora Prentice-Hall do Brasil Ltda., *Rio de Janeiro*

CONTENTS

PREFACE

This book tells you what to do about back pain. It tells you how to take care of it when it's there and how to keep it from coming back.

Back pain is not a simple problem. It is usually produced or aggravated by a combination of different factors. Every person's back pain is unique and changes from day to day. Even for the same person, therefore, the causes and proper treatment may change frequently.

Not everyone who wants to know about back pain has the same reason to learn. Some are experiencing the agonies of acute back pain. Some have just recovered from their first episode and are living in fear of a recurrence; some have chronic pain; some may have had no personal experience with back pain but need to know about it to help a patient, a relative, a client, or an employee.

My patients have made me appreciate the need for more teaching about back pain and back care for medical patients and for people before and after they are patients. In response to this need, my associates and I undertook the establishment of a back school. The idea of a back school was not new to us, but it is a fairly new concept in medical care—one that is explained further in this book. The biggest problem I faced in organizing a back school was the absence of an adequate manual that would be suitable as a text and reference book for all of the many different people with all of the many different back problems. Although there are many good books about back pain, none that are written for patients give thorough consideration to all of the varied causes and effects of back pain. More important, I felt that the presentations of many were in the language, or organized along the line of thinking, of doctors instead of patients.

I assembled the best information I could collect from what is written, from the teaching of colleagues, and from my personal experience in a way and in a language that I thought would be most helpful to the patients who would learn from it and to the doctors and therapists who would teach from it. I then submitted it to the trial of use by patients with many different back ailments and by nonpatients thought to be at risk of back pain.

The manual we have used in our back school explores the many factors that produce and aggravate back pain and the cycles by which one factor will provoke problems with another. It gives detailed descriptions of ways in which people can recognize the contributions made by each of these factors and the things they can do to improve each, and to establish positive cycles whereby improvement in one area increases success with efforts to improve another. All of those features of the manual have been preserved and expanded for this book. In addition, new sections have been added that provide better historical perspective, more analysis of some of the social consequences of back pain, more detailed and up-to-date information about medical and surgical care, and more specific information about how nonprofessionals can select and evaluate the need for professional care.

A lot of false hope, misadventure, and disappointment have been created by promises of one miracle cure for back pain. That has led to pessimism about back care in the minds of the public and many back pain sufferers. The idea that there is one cause and that there could be one simple remedy is faulty from its beginning. Once that idea is discarded and it is accepted that there are multiple factors involved, then there is real hope and cause for optimism.

The concept of holistic medicine—treating the whole person and not just the disease—has been much publicized in recent years. This book embraces that concept for two important reasons. One is that back pain usually has multiple causes. The other is that back pain often may be the signal of a more generalized health problem. Those who are excessively stressed, have poor health habits, get too little exercise, have poor diets, have little understanding of posture and body mechanics, and have lost their state of good fitness may break down first because of back pain, hypertension, heart disease, mental illness, or any number of other health problems. Just as back pain can be the avenue of exit from a state of health, the proper treatment of back pain can be the way to reenter good health and may prevent breakdown of other body functions.

The first step in overcoming a back problem is the willingness to work on it. It takes more than just willingness, however. It also takes confidence. Confidence comes from a thorough understanding of the problems and solutions. This book is written for those who are willing. It provides the information you need to understand and to take practical steps toward remedy.

Acknowledgments

This book contains a collection of many ideas from many different sources, all focused upon the problem of back pain. Few of the ideas are original; they are derived from the accumulated experiences of countless people who have contributed to the understanding of back disorders. The ideas have been contributed in the spirit of relieving human suffering to the medical literature and oral tradition to which I make collective acknowledgment.

The superb physicians with whom I practice at the Knoxville Orthopedic Clinic, the employees of the clinic, the staff of the Knoxville Back Care Center, and, most of all, our patients have stimulated me to be thorough and innovative in my practice. This stimulation led quite directly to the writing of this book.

My wife, Judy, and our children have helped me directly with many of the projects that contributed to the contents, with criticism of the writing, and with patience.

I owe thanks to Dennis Fawcett, my editor at Prentice-Hall, for encouragement and assistance. Thanks also to Suse Cioffi and the other members of the production staff at Prentice-Hall for making the publication of *Free Yourself from Neck Pain and Headache* such a pleasurable experience that I was encouraged to proceed with this book.

Cathy Shope, Toni Wyatt, Tommi Stubbs, Ron Phillips, John

Scofield, and Lutie Culver read early forms of the manuscript and made valuable suggestions. Bob Leggett and Dick Penner encouraged and assisted me in the effort to publish the material.

Faye Houston prepared the manuscript with a speed and accuracy that rivaled my word processor, all while she performed the many functions of a medical secretary with compassion and good humor. Her help has been invaluable, and her attitude has been inspiring.

To Alex, Amee, Josh, and Zach; to Maude; to Bo in her best year; and, as always, to Judy.

INTRODUCTION

Back pain is one of humanity's oldest problems. Records of medical practices from the earliest civilizations document that the search for a cure for back pain has held the attention of doctors throughout the ages.

It has been only in the last several decades that doctors have been able really to do anything to alter the course of most injuries and diseases. They have always been able to help recognize problems, to predict consequences, and to provide support and comfort. Sometimes the support and comfort were in the form of treatments that they at least implied would alter the course of the disease, and that implication gave patients and families hope for cures. But cures, when they came, in almost all instances were from natural causes, not from the treatments. Sometimes they were in spite of the treatments.

That helplessness of doctors to do anything that really altered disease has all changed in the past hundred years or so. Miracles of chemistry have provided us with drugs that cure diseases and tests that determine the needs for the precise type and dosage of drugs and that monitor their effects. Miracles of physics allow us safely to look into and through the nooks and crannies of the human body in search of areas of injury or disease that, once located, can be removed or repaired with a minimum of risk and pain.

What has all of this miraculous technology done for back pain? For some individuals, the miracles have come home. Back conditions that, in an earlier age, would have meant a lifetime of suffering have been completely cured by modern medicines or surgery for a few people. Those people and the doctors who have provided their care celebrate these triumphs. But those same doctors and other professionals who work with back pain know that, except for those few, the record does not look so good. With all of our technology and our ability to deliver miraculous cures to the few, the statistics show that, for the many, the back pain problem is worse than ever.

About 80 percent of people will have a major problem with back pain at some time in their lives. In the United States, the largest of the countries in which good statistics about back pain are kept, back pain is the number one cause of disability in people under age 45, and the figures are alarming. About 7 million Americans are down with back pain on any given day, 70 million have had at least one episode of severe low back pain, and each year 15 million go to doctors because of back pain.

Besides the $5 billion a year that Americans spend on medical care for low back pain, the economic impact is enormous. Every year, 52 out of every 1000 workers will have a work-related back injury, 18 of them will be off from work for longer than a month, and four never will return to work. Almost 100 million work days are lost in the United States each year because of back pain. About 33 percent of the workers' compensation dollar and 60 percent of long-term disability payment money go toward back injuries. Statistics from other developed countries don't look any better than those from the United States. In some respects, some are worse.

The 200,000 or so operations done in the United States each year to try to cure back pain don't seem to make much of a dent in the statistics. Neither do all of the medicines and other treatments offered as cures for back pain by various medical specialists, physical therapists, biofeedback therapists, hypnotists, acupuncturists, psychologists, chiropractors, pharmacists, nutritionists, health and exercise leaders, nurses, and others. And the social impact continues to be enormous in spite of the efforts of insurance adjusters, lawyers, safety officers, vocational rehabilitation counselors, social workers, and all those involved in the effort to keep back pain from ruining lives and obstructing productivity.

As the ones who control the technical power to effect predictable and understandable cures in the few cases that lend themselves to it, physicians are looked to for leadership in overcoming the ubiquitous back pain problem. Just as the physicians of centuries past knew in their hearts that they didn't possess the tools needed really to cure anything, physicians today know that their skills with drugs and surgery will really cure only a few and will not appreciably improve the alarming statistics that reflect the personal and economic suffering wrought by back conditions.

For physicians to approach the huge specter of back pain and to be effective in dealing with it, they must go beyond their roles as technical experts and return to what the best of them always were—teachers. The word *doctor* is derived from the Latin *docere,* which means "to teach."

Most people can cure and prevent their own back pain. If they were taught how, that would improve those statistics more than all of the surgery and medicine ever will. Most people don't need specialists and professionals to manage their back pain problems. If those who do could understand more about back pain, they would be able to choose what professionals they need and when, they would be better patients, and they would get better results.

Back pain is not a simple problem. It is too bad that it doesn't have a simple cause and a simple cure, but it doesn't. Unless we accept that, we are doomed to go off on one tangent after another, to one type of professional after another, trying one gimmick after another—all failures because none accounts for the whole picture. Each aspect of the problem has the potential to provoke other aspects of back pain, so cycles occur that recreate and intensify the problem in spite of well-intentioned efforts along one line or another.

Once the whole picture is painted and all of the details of back pain are understood, lasting progress can be made. Then, good cycles can be created whereby improvement along one line makes improvement of other aspects easier and more likely.

This book describes the many aspects of a back pain problem, explaining the ways in which back pain is caused by stresses of posture, work, and play; muscle weakness; joint stiffness; poor nutrition; psychological reactions; lack of general fitness; misunderstandings of the influences of compensation and legal factors; misinterpretation of the relationship between back pain and sex; misuse of drugs and alcohol; and ignorance of body mechanics. The explanations are accompanied by simple instructions about what you can do, on your own, to relieve the pain.

First in the book—and, for many people, first in importance—is a chapter on first aid measures that you can take to relieve back pain when it occurs. This is important, not just for the immediate relief it provides, but also because it alleviates fear. For those who have had severe back pain, one of the greatest problems is overcoming the fear of recurrence. That fear keeps many people from trying things that would make them better. Knowing how to manage effectively the occurrence of pain helps alleviate that fear and is a natural first step toward overcoming the problem.

This book is comprehensive. It does not have much technical, detailed medical information with case histories, x rays, and descriptions of unusual diseases. Those are things that need to be understood by doctors who are providing the technical management of certain back pain problems. The book, then, is comprehensive in the sense that it tries to explore every aspect of the back pain problem that relates to people who are trying to care for themselves. In many places, the exploration is very detailed where those details seem necessary to the understanding of self-care.

This book does provide a lot of medical information—information about surgery and disc injections, sophisticated x-ray tests, anatomy, and medications. This is presented to provide an understanding for those who have had or may have medical treatment for a back problem. If you are such a person, this material should make you a better and more successful patient.

The book provides more information about workers' compensation and the legal, social, and psychological aspects of back pain than is available in other self-care books. All of the professionals who deal with back pain problems know what a big role these factors play. Because they are regarded as personal and difficult to talk about, however, they are often given little mention in material offered to patients. These are not just problems for society, though; they cause a lot of personal suffering for back pain patients.

This book is written for people with back pain. It uses language that nonprofessionals understand. It approaches the subjects by giving first consideration and emphasis to those things that are most important to back pain sufferers. It is also written for professionals who care for people with back pain. All professionals have a tunnel-vision perspective on back pain because they must address their specialized skills to one or another aspect of the problem. The comprehensive nature of this book allows them to broaden their views and to see the whole picture from the patient's perspective. The book was derived originally from a manual for therapists to use in teaching back care to patients, and it still lends itself ideally to that use.

Because the book is comprehensive and detailed, it serves well as a reference guide to be consulted about specific aspects of back pain when the need arises. I suggest, however, that those with back pain read it straight through once and then use it as a reference. Only by reading it straight through does the whole picture emerge. The development of the whole picture with whole remedies is the theme of the book.

1
FIRST AID

First aid for back pain means self-application of simple treatments to relieve acute back pain. The treatments must be easily and quickly available. They should be safe and effective. They should not require professional help.

There are many treatments that have been applied to people with back pain. There are surgical operations for back pain. Many medicines are used to relieve pain, relax muscles, or reduce inflammation. Direct injections of drugs and coagulation devices into many different sites of origin of back pain are in use. The back may be heated, cooled, stimulated by sound waves and electrical impulses, massaged, twisted, stretched, pulled upon, and manipulated in numerous ways. All sorts of things can be rubbed in, plastered upon, or bound around the back. The mind's control over the body may be tapped by such treatments as psychotherapy, hypnosis, and biofeedback.

All of these treatments have worked for some people at some time. None of them works for everyone all of the time. All have a common factor. They all require some expert, some practitioner, to do something to the person with the back pain.

This book will teach self-care of your back. By correct application of the techniques described, back pain should diminish in both severity and frequency. There still may be times when back pain flares up and more than preventive measures are needed. During those times, first aid measures, self-applied, usually will solve the problem.

Confidence that you can handle your own back care even when problems arise is an important part of solving the difficulties caused by back pain. Fear of back pain sometimes becomes a worse problem than the actual pain. You can learn to rid yourself of that fear by learning not only how to prevent the pain but also to care for it when it occurs.

Rest Position

You will learn about the effects of different body positions on the low back. First, you should learn the position that is most likely to relieve back pain—the rest position. (See Figure 1.)

Find a chair or a couch at a height that allows you to lie on the floor with your legs on the seat. You also could use large pillows stacked up for this.

Your hips should be touching the floor, and your legs should be completely at rest with the knees and hips bent at a right angle. Use a small, flat pillow for your head if that is comfortable. Remove eyeglasses and bulky jewelry. Loosen neckties and tight clothing. Close your eyes and mouth lightly. Let your jaw, tongue, and mouth relax, and let your forehead go smooth.

This is the rest position. From it you may do the relaxation exercises that you will learn later in the book. Simply resting in this position for a few minutes will relieve most back pain.

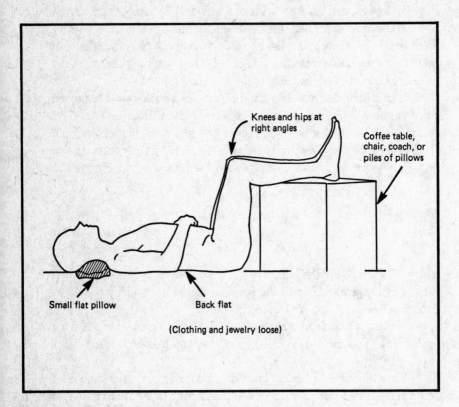

Knees and hips at right angles

Coffee table, chair, coach, or piles of pillows

Small flat pillow

Back flat

(Clothing and jewelry loose)

FIGURE 1. The Rest Position.

When you have done something to reinjure your back or set off a painful muscle spasm, you may use ice massage to relieve the spasm. Keep a foam or paper cup of water frozen in your freezer. Peel off the top two or three centimeters of the cup. Lie on your side with one pillow between your knees and a smaller pillow under your head. Massage for up to ten minutes in the area of the pain. You may do this yourself or, if you have willing help, you may lie on your stomach over a pillow and have someone give you a massage.

As soon as you have finished the ice massage, lie on your back. With your hands, grasp the backs of your thighs just above the knees, and pull your knees to your chest. Hold this position for three to five minutes to stretch the low back muscles after the ice massage.

In most circumstances, heat and cold act as opposite forces. The effects of the two on sore muscles, however, may be very similar. The changes produced by ice may penetrate a little deeper, and because the surface discomfort limits the time it can be tolerated, ice may be a little safer.

Ice is usually more effective when the pain has come on abruptly and is accompanied by muscle spasm. Heat, properly applied, can be very soothing and can help with mobilization of tight muscles and joints, especially if the problem has come on more slowly and has been present for more than a day or two. The back is much like other areas of the body in this regard; sprains, strains, and bruises that have just occurred are best treated with ice, whereas tight, stiff, sore areas of longer duration are often soothed by heat.

Sitting or standing in a shower with hot water bathing the sore areas is a safe and effective means of heat application. Putting a towel over the sore area so that the shower water hits the towel maintains an even, comfortable heat.

Heating pads, if used, should be set at low intensity. Prolonged applications of high temperatures cook the skin, producing a mottled appearance. To avoid skin injury, it is best to alternate 20 minutes of contact on with one hour off. The sensation of heat may be perpetuated by applying mentholated balms.

Massage and Acupressure

The muscles of the lower back are deeply situated, and the structures responsible for the pain may be even deeper. It is difficult, therefore, especially for overweight people, for massage to be directly effective for low back pain. There may be indirect effects of massage that are quite helpful, however.

Pain states may be perpetuated by cycles of reactions wherein the underlying anatomic abnormality becomes only one factor, sometimes not the most important factor. One such cycle involves the muscles and the nerves that control the muscles.

Direct finger massage of tight or tender muscles may help break these pain cycles. The massage may be effective even at sites quite remote from the primary problem. The most common sites for such a phenomenon are at the motor points of muscles. The motor points are the action sites in muscles where the nerves fire the electrochemical shot that leads to muscle contraction. Motor points generally conform closely to favored sites for acupuncture. A variation of acupuncture—acupressure—is a massage technique that can be safely self-applied.

You may have found your own trigger spots, tender foci in the muscles of the back, hip, or leg that may cause the pain to radiate when they are irritated. If gently but firmly pressed, they may cause the pain to be relieved. These, too, are likely to conform to areas of motor points.

Acupressure can be self-applied in certain locations. It is necessary in some spots, and preferable in all, to have someone else do it for you. It is quite safe and simple, so it need not require a professional to try it.

Since most acupressure sites are on the posterior (back) side, it is usually best for the recipient to lie face down with the hips bent over a pillow or two and with a pillow under the feet. Comfort and relaxation are important for both the subject and the helper.

Use the tip of the finger or thumb directly over the point, making small, circular motions at a rate of about two per second. Maintain continuous contact. Continuous pressure should be exerted in that spot for at least three and up to five minutes.

Common sites for effective acupressure are in the muscles along the side of the spine about two finger-widths to the side of the midline at the level of the navel, in the buttock muscles about a hand's-breadth below the top of the pelvic bone and the same distance out from the midline of the lower back, in the midportion of the back of the thigh along the inside where your fingertips would reach if you were to grasp the midthigh as though to lift the leg with the opposite hand, and about a hand's-width above the bend of the knee where your fingertips would reach if you were to grasp your thigh above the knee as though to lift your leg with the arm on the same side. There are also several motor points below the knee that usually can be localized by trial and error.

Body Traction and Mobilization

Gradual stretching and positioning of the body may apply a traction pull to certain areas of the back and relieve pain. Different techniques work for different people and may vary in effectiveness for the same person at different times. All should be gradual and gentle and should be limited to about five minutes at first, working up to no more than 15 minutes. Longer duration with some of these techniques could have harmful results.

A healthy back depends upon the balanced, normal function of the front of the spine with the back of the spine. The structures toward the front of the spine, called the anterior elements, include the discs. Those toward the back of the spine, the posterior elements, include the facet joints. Later in this book, you will learn more about the anatomy of these structures, and you will learn specific techniques to improve the functions of both anterior and posterior structures. Most people find that they have more problem with the function of either one or the other of these anterior and posterior elements.

You will learn exercises that emphasize the area of your greatest need for improved flexibility and strength. Likewise, if back pain flares up, you will want to apply first aid to relieve whichever of the structures is causing you the most pain. Some people will experience flares of pain from front side structures one time and from the back side another time so it may require some trial and error.

Generally, people who have pain from the posterior structures do best to position themselves with the lower back bent forward (flexed). People with this type of pain usually have more pain while standing or walking downhill and are relieved when sitting and leaning over a desk. First aid posturing begins with the rest position and can be extended by placing a pillow under the buttocks.

Many people who have pain from the posterior structures have more trouble on one side than the other. Doing a side stretch may provide relief from this one-sided pain. For the side stretch, lie with the painful side up and with a pillow or two under the other side between the ribs and the pelvis. (See Figure 2a.)

Some people, usually those who experience pain from the posterior structures, have periodic, sudden, painful catches in the lower back. Some have experienced sudden relief of these catches by accidental twisting motions or by purposeful manipulations by chiropractors or other professionals who treat by manipulation.

There is a distinction between mobilization and manipulation. With mobilization, a prolonged or repeated gentle effort is made to stretch the part to gain full motion. Manipulation adds a sudden, forceful effort applied at the extreme of what is achieved by mobilization. Almost all catches and cricks can be relieved as effectively and more safely by mobilization without the need for quickly applied additional force.

There is an effective and generally safe way to apply mobilization to relieve catches and sudden occurrences of posterior element back pain. If you have severe sciatic pain that radiates down the leg below the knee, you should not use this technique and you should not allow yourself to be treated by forceful manipulations that involve twisting. The technique—the side stretch roll—works best for those with low back

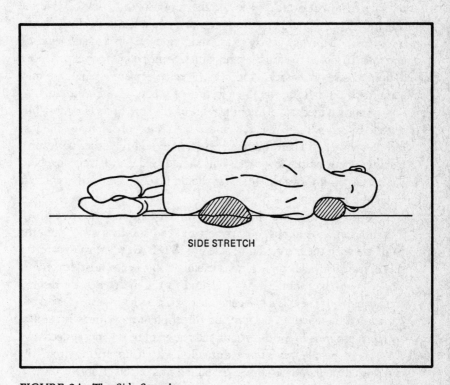

FIGURE 2A. The Side Stretch.

pain that is greater on one side, is aggravated by attempts to stand straight and lean back, and does not radiate below the knee.

The side stretch roll begins in the same position as the side stretch, with the painful side up. It is usually easiest to do this on the edge of a firm bed or couch. Slowly pull the top knee up to the chest and allow the top hip to roll forward. Then let the top arm roll backward at the shoulder. There should be a mild, twisting strain felt in the lower back, but no pain. You may gently rotate and jiggle the top arm and leg back and forth to loosen the muscles and joints. Some people may experience a popping noise or sensation followed by relief of pain. Relief also may come with no definite sound or feeling of a pop. (See Figure 2b.)

Another method of mobilization of the low back is done while seated. By straddling a chair, you can lock your pelvis into a straight, forward position. Then roll one arm forward and the other backward, placing a twist on the low back. This should be done with the low back flat and leaning forward a little. It should be done gradually, without sudden jerking motions.

With the side stretch, the side stretch roll, and the seated back mobilization, it is almost always best to bend and turn away from the pain. Lie with the most painful side up. When seated, turn toward the side of least pain. These directions usually result in the least discomfort while doing the mobilizations and lead to the most effective results. Occasionally, if there is more generalized pain and stiffness, it is best to get started by whatever posture and direction of movement is painless and then progress to the directions you reason to be the most effective.

Some people have more difficulty with pain arising from the anterior elements of the spine. In some forms of this problem, flexion bending can make the back hurt worse. Generally, these people have more pain when sitting in a forward-leaning or slouched position. They hurt worse when they have to bend forward or twist. They may feel better when they are walking about with the back straight. People who have pain radiating down the back of the leg to below the knee are usually in this group, though many people in this group do not have such sciatic pain.

If you have anterior pain, you may be relieved by mobilization in

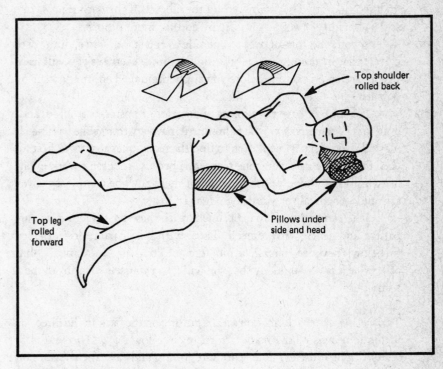

FIGURE 2B. The Side Stretch Roll.

extension. Begin with five to ten minutes of lying flat on the stomach (prone). Follow that by gradually propping the upper body up on the elbows. Assist with pillows under the chest to take pressure off the arms.

If this type of extension posturing comes easily and seems to help, you may progress at subsequent sessions by doing up to ten push-offs, keeping the pelvis down flat and smoothly pushing the upper body up for a second or two by straightening the elbows. If this technique is safe and successful for you, extend it by adding more pillows.

If you tend to pull over to one side as you stand, you should try to correct that by doing the side-gliding flexibility exercises you will learn in the section on exercise before you apply prolonged effort at extension posturing.

Few people have pure forms of anterior or posterior trouble, and, even for the same person, the pain source may vary from time to time. It may take some experimentation to find the techniques that work best for you. Don't give up on any one technique because it doesn't work in one or two tries, and don't push too vigorously at any one until it is proven safe and beneficial for you by gradual trial.

It is generally safe to experiment with these techniques if you are patient and gentle with yourself. Those with sciatic pain, down the leg to below the knee, should avoid forceful, twisting movements, but otherwise it is very unlikely that you will harm yourself with any of these techniques.

Traction Devices. Back traction means pulling on the back in the direction of the long axis of the body, stretching the low back. The idea is to stretch tight muscles, pull apart sore joints, and take the pressure off painful discs. Some of the techniques just described show how these things can be done by body positioning. Some gadgetry is available for home use to assist in achieving these goals.

The traction device most people are familiar with is bed traction, applied through a pelvic sling with weights hung off the end of the bed. This type of traction has long been in common use for back treatment in hospitals. In this system, the weights have to be light enough that they do not injure the skin, yet heavy enough to overcome not only muscle pull and ligament tension but also the body weight friction against the bed. It can't be done perfectly. Nonetheless, it works to relieve pain for many people.

Bed traction doesn't work by successfully rearranging the anatomy. It works because it relaxes the muscles by giving a gentle pull in a comfortable position and because it exerts a comforting contact pressure around the low back and abdomen. It makes bed rest easier for some.

Bed traction can be applied at home. A pelvic sling, ropes, weights, and suspension apparatus can be purchased at most orthopedic supply houses. Costs are not exorbitant. A doctor's prescription is sometimes necessary.

Bed traction is safe for most people to apply and leave on for hours at a time. The amount of weight that can be tolerated in this type of traction is usually around 12 to 15 pounds. Those who must avoid any increase in pelvic and leg vein pressure—such as pregnant women, phlebitis patients, and anyone prone to blood clotting for any reason— should not apply traction to themselves.

In order to exert enough force to really pull on the structures of the lower back, the body weight must be used to exert the pull. This requires such force that the traction usually can be tolerated only for brief periods.

A very simple and inexpensive way to apply body weight traction to the lower back is by using crutches. It is hard to suspend the body from crutches for long periods, and care must be taken not to bruise the nerves that pass through the armpit. Most of the weight should be taken on the hands and forearms. The physical effort required for walking with crutches may even aggravate the back problem for those who are not strong in their arms. If you are skilled with crutches and strong in your arms, however, you may use crutches to relieve some of the stress of weight bearing and exert an intermittent traction pull on the low back. This is meant only as a first aid measure and not as a means of adapting to chronic back pain.

Suspension frames for short-duration (less than 30 minutes) heavy traction are also available for home use. You lie on the floor and pull your hips up off the floor with a rope that runs through a ratchet pulley on the frame and down to a pelvic sling. Most of the work goes toward overcoming body weight so that little additional pull is placed across the entire spine. A strong forward pull into flexion of the low back is exerted. The device may be helpful for posterior element pain, but, at least in theory, it could aggravate certain anterior problems.

There has been much recent attention, mostly because of commercial marketing, focused on gravity traction apparatus such as inversion boots. By hanging upside down by the legs or feet, a strong traction force can be exerted across the lower back. This is not a new idea. There are, in fact, pictorial records of its use in ancient times. It has been carefully studied over many years in some modern medical settings, but it has never achieved wide medical acceptance. The Food and Drug Administration has issued a warning that advertisers should not claim that these products have medical benefits. Reluctance to recommend such a device for general use comes from concerns about the ability of the unathletic, the injured, and those in pain to protect themselves adequately when getting into and out of the device; the possible harmful effects on other joints and musculoskeletal structures; and the side effects from circulatory changes in the brain and the eyes. Elderly people and people with hypertension, retinal detachment, hiatal hernia, a history of stroke or other brain disorders, and people taking anti-inflammatory drugs or blood thinners should not try inversion traction. For those who have been guided in the use of such devices, who have proven through trial that it is safe and effective for them, and who have no special reasons to fear circulatory complications, it may be an effective means of overcoming muscle spasm in the lower back.

Neither gravity traction nor any other means of traction or manipulation will return a ruptured disc to its rightful location or otherwise produce a healthful, permanent reordering of the anatomy. These methods are meant to deal with the secondary effects complicating an underlying low back disorder. They are first aid techniques for symptom relief. They are not treatment methods meant to effect permanent cures. You understand the wisdom of keeping the methods as safe, inexpensive, and uncomplicated as possible. That makes other first aid measures preferable to the use of traction devices.

Medicines

Excessive reliance on medication can obstruct the effort to get to the source of some of the important aspects of a back problem. The idea that medicine can cure back pain the way penicillin cures a strep throat is incorrect.

There is no doubt, though, that some medications can help with some back pains, particularly if the back pain is acute. Fortunately, some very effective medicines are available without prescription and can qualify as first aid, self-care treatment.

Aspirin is one of the most effective pain-relieving and anti-inflammatory medications. To help control acute back pain, it is best to take aspirin on a regular schedule, four times a day, and not to wait to take it until the pain is most severe. Eight to 12 aspirin per day is the usual effective dosage. Your pharmacist can help you select coated aspirin to help avoid stomach upset. If you have an ulcer, problems with blood clotting or intestinal bleeding, or any history of allergy to aspirin, you should not take aspirin.

Acetaminophen does not have the anti-inflammatory properties, but it is an effective pain reliever and does not carry as much worry about side effects as does aspirin. It may be taken in addition to aspirin if you can tolerate both.

Back Supports

Braces, corsets, belts, or binders don't cure back pain and are usually not helpful for long-term use. A properly fitting device that gives additional abdominal and back support can be very helpful for short-term use, however. Frequently, they can improve function pending the long-range benefits of exercise and other curative measures.

Braces with heavy metal or plastic parts are meant more to restrict motion than to give real support. They are generally used only when prescribed by a physician for a specific problem that requires extraordinary stability or an attempt to position the spine rigidly.

Some people become accustomed to the use of corsets for back pain and support. Most people find corsets too cumbersome and too much trouble.

Anything that makes contact around the painful area in back and puts pressure through the abdomen in front makes acute back pain feel better. The simplest, least expensive, and best tolerated of these devices are elastic bands that have self-adhering closures in front so that you may wrap one quite easily around your waist, pull it together in front, and conceal it with hardly a notice beneath your clothing. These are available in various widths and sold as elastic abdominal binders, rib belts, or lumbosacral belts. Some of the lumbosacral belts are designed to place a pressure pad in back and don't give much abdominal support in front. Most people find that the wider devices that give a lot of abdominal support are much more effective in relieving acute back pain.

One disadvantage of simple elastic devices is that they tend to wrinkle and roll after they have been worn for a while. A modification that does better in that regard and provides a little additional support without being too restrictive and uncomfortable is the reinforced binder. Metal staves or a molded plastic insert give partial rigidity across the back.

The simple, unreinforced binder has some major advantages if you are not already comfortable with some other form of support. It is inexpensive and does not require a doctor's prescription. It can be rolled up and kept in a drawer, glove compartment, or suitcase with ease. You can find them at most drug stores. They are effective enough in relieving pain and improving function in the presence of pain that they are recommended to anyone with a back pain problem. They should not be worn in bed or during prolonged sitting, such as during a long automobile ride. They are meant to support the back and abdomen while you are standing and walking during periods of acute pain. They are first aid devices for temporary use, not a substitute for the exercises needed to manage chronic pain and prevent the occurrence of pain.

2
POSTURE

Posture means the attitude or position in which the body is held. The posture of the body has considerable influence upon the stresses that bear on the lower back. Since the low back is near the center of the body, it can be thought of as the axis around which the body rotates. Variations in the posture of the other body parts change the forces that act on that axis of rotation.

The ancient masters of karate and other similar disciplines placed great emphasis on spinal posture. They regarded the lower back and pelvis as being near the center of the soul. Students were required to spend many months developing proper posture before advancing to other aspects of those arts. Though the reasons are different, many of the teachings about posture for modern people with back pain are similar to those ancient instructions.

A healthy lower back depends upon a balance created by strong muscles and flexible joints around a spine held in proper posture. Posture stresses are different in standing, sitting, and lying positions. They also may be different for different people depending upon body build and any variations from normal spinal anatomy.

Normal and Abnormal Low Back Posture

The normal lumbar spine has a back-to-front curvature. Looking from the side, there is a concavity or sway just above the belt line. This curvature is called the lumbar lordosis. Some lordosis is normal and helps put the body in the best functional position for many activities.

If too much of the strain of weight bearing is absorbed by allowing the back to sway into excess lordosis, pain can result. Excessive lordosis or too much stress in a lordotic position may narrow the spaces between the vertebrae of the lower back. The spinal nerves pass through these spaces on their way out to the hips and legs. If the spaces are narrowed, the nerves may be pinched and their circulation impaired.

The vertebrae join together on their back sides at the facet joints. The contact areas of these joints are rather small. Excessive lordosis increases the forces across these little joints and makes it difficult for them to allow bending and turning movements without pain.

If you stand with your back to a wall and touch your hips and shoulder blades to the wall, you can slide your hand between your lower back and the wall. The space that is available for your hand is a measure of the space created by your lordosis. If you then tilt your hips and pull in your abdomen, you can flatten your back against the wall. This is called reducing the lordosis. The movement that reduces the lordosis is called a pelvic tilt.

The posture achieved by tilting the pelvis to reduce the lordosis results in less stress on the discs, joints, and nerves of the lower back. Tilting the pelvis makes the base upon which the spine is supported flatter and more stable. By pulling in the abdomen, you support the front of your spine. Maintenance of that posture while standing will relieve and prevent many forms of back pain.

Most people have been taught about posture since childhood. It is not always easy to do something correctly just because you've been told how. Sometimes nagging a child about standing up straight even gets in the way of a mature understanding of the importance of good back posture. It requires some mental effort to break old habits and learn new ways. It also requires some physical effort, because more muscular energy is needed to stand properly than to let it sag.

There are strong ligaments across the front of the hip joint from the pelvis to the thigh bone. If you let the pelvis roll forward and let the low back sag into lordosis, you can lean on these ligaments and remain standing the lazy way without using your muscles to hold your back straight and your pelvis tilted. The price you pay for this laziness is excessive wear and tear on the lower back. The anulus ligaments that support the discs are kept under stretch, and the little facet joints must endure extraordinary forces.

Most people who stand with their backs sagging and bellies hanging over the belt do so for more reasons than just laziness. Posture is influenced by other factors besides muscular efficiency. Heredity and the learning experiences of early childhood certainly play roles in the development of posture habits. Many people stand and move in ways similar to those of their parents.

Posture is one way in which the body reflects inner emotions. We stand and move according to how we feel. It is usually easy to determine who is winning a tennis match by watching the way the players stand and walk between points. People who feel like they are losing all the time stand and move as though, like Atlas, they have the weight of the world on their shoulders.

Some people maintain a forward-stooped posture, with neck forward and down and shoulders slumped as a holdover from the psychological adjustment of adolescence. During the years of rapid growth, many people don't want to stand up straight. They want to blend in and be unnoticed. This may be a particular problem for people who grow very tall or for girls who develop large breasts. Attempts to conceal height or buxomness may lead to habitual bad posture.

The body position that signals being afraid and ready either to fight to defend oneself or to flee to safety is the crouched, shortened posture. Strength and feelings of security and confidence are associated with standing tall.

Besides reflecting feelings, posture is a signal to the world of how you expect to be treated. The sagging, weighted, downtrodden posture demands no respect and invites further abuse.

Posture, therefore, is a reflection of several things: the status of ligaments and muscles, feelings generated by past experience, expectations of the future, and habit. All of these things can't be changed easily or rapidly, but posture can be improved immediately and steps can be initiated to ensure continued improvement.

What to Do About Standing Posture

Begin by learning the pelvic tilt. Maintain it as much as you can. Pretend there is a weight on top of your head that you must push up without letting your heels leave the floor. To do this, you must straighten your spine.

When you feel the sensation of making your spine straighter and longer, of getting taller, you will feel the interdependence of the various parts of your spine. Good low back posture depends upon good posture of the head, neck, and shoulders. The head should be back over the shoulders with the neck straight. The shoulders should be drawn back so that the shoulder blades are held near each other in back. This doesn't mean that an extreme, military-brace posture should be held. If you pull into that extreme posture and then relax by about 25 percent, you will achieve a good compromise that is both comfortable and healthful.

Practice the pelvic tilt and getting taller by combining simple exercises with some mental images. Stand flat against the wall in a fully relaxed, slumped attitude. Feel the space between the wall and the curve of your lower back. Now think of a wire attached to the top of your head, pulling you up straight, taller. Feel the curve flatten from your lower back, your shoulder blades come together as your shoulders are pulled back, and your neck get straighter and longer as your head comes up higher. Now walk away from the wall, maintaining this posture and the image of the wire pulling you up taller.

A similar exercise is to balance a book on top of your head while standing against a wall. Try to walk away from the wall and keep the book balanced on your head. You will find that you are much more successful with this if you maintain proper spinal posture.

Another useful image is to think of a third eye at the front of the lower neck, about where the knot of a necktie would be. You must stand and move in a way that allows the third eye to see well at all times. That is not possible if you allow your spine to slump and your shoulders and neck to droop.

You can recall these images whenever you catch yourself falling into bad posture. You won't have to go through the whole exercise starting from the wall. The images help you to recall instantly all of the aspects of good posture without having to stop to think through the positions of various body parts.

If the muscles used to maintain good posture are very strong, it is much easier to avoid excess lordosis and spinal slumping. One step to good posture, therefore, is to do muscle strengthening exercises. This is especially important for those whose abdominal muscles have been weakened by pregnancies or abdominal surgery, but it is important for everyone who is trying to escape back pain. Exercise to strengthen muscles is an absolute necessity for good posture. It takes a long time to strengthen muscles, though, so you must be patient.

The amount of weight that is carried in the abdomen is an important aspect of posture for many people. The volume and weight of fat in the abdominal wall and within the abdominal cavity are major determinants of the stresses placed on the lower spine. They also influence the efficiency of the trunk muscles that must help handle those stresses. For those who are overweight, losing abdominal fat is a slow but important part of the solution to back pain resulting from excessive lumbar stress in lordosis.

While working at muscle strengthening and abdominal weight reduction, it may help to hold some of the abdominal weight artificially with a wide belt, corset, binder, or brace. Dependence on appliances without proper attention to other factors can make things worse in the long run, but using an appliance as a temporary device during times of special stress may help to maintain proper posture.

When standing with both feet together and flat on the floor, there is a tendency for the lower back to drift into too much lordosis. If you simply place one foot in front of the other, it helps a little. If the forward foot can be lifted and placed on a small stool, shelf, or rail, the tendency to excess lordosis and, with it, the tendency to develop back pain are much reduced. If you are able to rest a hand, forearm, or elbow at elbow level, you further diminish back stress.

Standing at and leaning over a typical tavern bar with a foot rail is an example of an ideal position for avoiding back pain while standing. It was no accident that innkeepers discovered that tired workers would patronize their taverns longer when such a provision was made to keep their backs from hurting. The innkeepers also learned that back strain could be further alleviated if they provided a high stool for periodic sitting. Others need to discover and employ the same standing aids at their work and in their homes.

Old habits should not be changed abruptly. Awareness of bad habits and knowledge of what constitutes good posture, however, will lead you to make repeated little adjustments that eventually have a beneficial result. Changing bad habits is a matter of awareness and a commitment to keep making adjustments in the right direction and never to slip back into old, harmful habits. It takes the body and the mind some time to adapt. The continued effort to improve is the important thing.

Why Change?

Changing posture habits is not easy even though you can make a great temporary improvement with a single effort. Posture may be inherited or learned from an early age. The psychological aspects of posture and body language may take a long while to adjust. Physical adaptations have occurred that make it physically easier to do it the old way.

These factors must be balanced by the desire to relieve or prevent the pain and other symptoms caused by the old posture habits. It is very tempting to seek the solution in some pill, manipulation, or other solution that someone offers. No one else, however, can solve the problems that you create with bad posture habits.

One of the problems with changing posture is that it may require more muscular effort at first. Posture habits become lazy habits. That is part of the reason why changing posture habits may seem unnatural and a lot of effort at first.

What is gained, of course, is freedom from the pain and effects of progressive unhealthful changes in the spine. Healthy use of muscles is good for them. They can be conditioned to accept extra work without discomfort.

The social and psychological rewards of a strong, upright presence can be considered bonuses added to the relief from pain and the maintenance of the integrity of the spine.

Sitting Posture—Maintaining the Lordosis

The best sitting posture for most people requires that the natural sway of the lower back be preserved and supported—that the lordosis be maintained. At first, this may seem contradictory to what has been said about the value of reducing the lordosis. The advice to flatten the lower back applies to standing, walking, and reaching. The stresses from sitting are quite different.

The people who have the most trouble from sitting or from their sitting habits need to learn to avoid the tendency to sit with the lumbar spine excessively flexed. Lumbar flexion, the forward bending of the lower back, is not likely to occur to excess while standing. It is, however, a very common excess of faulty, slouched sitting.

Remember that a balanced spine stays healthy. Excess flexion posture can cause trouble just as excess lordosis causes trouble. Certain individuals have more problems from one than from the other, but poor posture habits in either direction can cause difficulties. The trouble is not always immediately apparent. The changes that occur in the structures of the lower back after excess flexion, such as from prolonged slouched sitting or forward bending, may cause pain later when standing or applying different stresses to the back.

It is best to sit with your feet comfortably flat on the floor. The knees and hips should be at right angles to the floor and to each other. A variation on this, helpful to some people, is to begin with the hips and knees at right angles and then raise the knees slightly by placing a small stool under one or both feet. The stool can be moved when you prepare to stand. Though this knees-up position is usually comfortable to the back, it is best not to use a low armchair to achieve it, because getting into and out of such a chair may be too stressful.

You should sit in chairs with back rests which contour well to your lumbar lordosis. (See Figure 3.) Straight-back chairs or supports adjusted too high so that there is a forward push on the upper back and no restful support to the lumbar area may cause back pain. A sitting surface which is comfortable and positions you to receive the lumbar support is equally important.

If you must sit in a chair without adequate lumbar support, take a towel and roll it up to a size that gives you comfortable lumbar support, tape or tie it to stay that size, and place it in the hollow between the low back and the back of the chair.

Chairs with armrests are best. A little of your weight can be taken through the armrest while sitting. More importantly, the armrest can substantially unload the stresses on the lower back when you change position or get into or out of the chair. The features of work chairs, stools, and other sitting surfaces are discussed in greater detail in Chapter 3.

Don't be afraid to move around in your chair. Children know they are more comfortable if they wiggle in chairs, but they are taught to sit still. Adults have retained those learned inhibitions about wiggling, sometimes to the disadvantage of their backs. Older people have traditionally returned to movement while sitting by using rocking chairs. President John F. Kennedy treated his bad back with a rocking chair that became one of his trademarks.

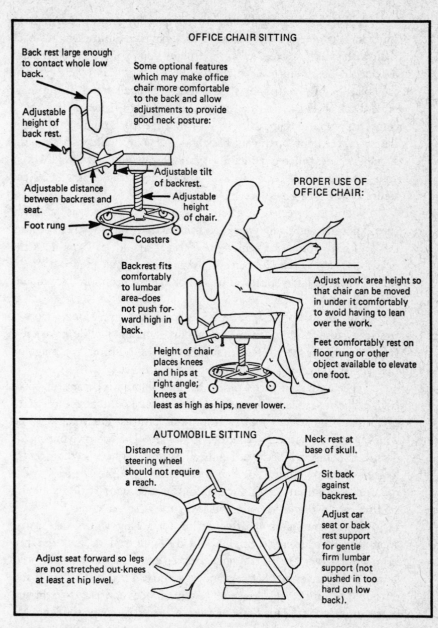

OFFICE CHAIR SITTING

Back rest large enough to contact whole low back.

Adjustable height of back rest.

Some optional features which may make office chair more comfortable to the back and allow adjustments to provide good neck posture:

Adjustable tilt of backrest.

Adjustable height of chair.

Adjustable distance between backrest and seat.

Foot rung

Coasters

Backrest fits comfortably to lumbar area–does not push forward high in back.

Height of chair places knees and hips at right angle; knees at least as high as hips, never lower.

PROPER USE OF OFFICE CHAIR:

Adjust work area height so that chair can be moved in under it comfortably to avoid having to lean over the work.

Feet comfortably rest on floor rung or other object available to elevate one foot.

AUTOMOBILE SITTING

Distance from steering wheel should not require a reach.

Neck rest at base of skull.

Sit back against backrest.

Adjust car seat or back rest support for gentle firm lumbar support (not pushed in too hard on low back).

Adjust seat forward so legs are not stretched out-knees at least at hip level.

FIGURE 3. Sitting Posture.

A short exercise that demonstrates the differences in sitting postures can help determine your ideal sitting posture. Sit in a straight-back chair with your legs stretched out in front of you. Your feet should touch only at the heels, and your knees should be lower than your hips. The only places where your body should touch the chair are at the hips and upper back. Feel the slouched, flexed position of the lower back. Now completely reverse that position. Pull your feet back under you so they are flat on the floor. Arch your back and pull your shoulders back so the shoulder blades pinch together in the middle of your upper back. Throw your head and neck back so that you look up at the ceiling. Feel the return of the lordosis to your lower back.

This overcorrected position causes too much lordosis, and you should not hold it. Bring your head back so that you face straight ahead but still have your head centered over your shoulders. Now relax the whole position about 20 percent from the extreme. Your shoulders should be back, and your lower back should have a comfortable amount of lordosis.

Maintenance of even the most ideal position for very long periods of time can cause trouble. If you shift about, stand for a while, take a few steps, stretch, or spend a few minutes in the rest position, you may find that you tolerate long periods of sitting much better

If you cannot sit with a proper amount of lordosis because of a poor chair or the need to lean forward over a desk, you should stand every 30 to 60 minutes and stretch your back into full lordosis. Put your hands on your buttocks. First rotate your pelvis forward. Then throw your shoulders, head, and neck backward and arch your lower back so that you are looking at the ceiling. You can repeat this ten times in less than a minute. One minute of this stretching for each hour of flexed sitting posture can save a lot of pain and lost time from backache.

Before you stand up after sitting for a long while, take a few seconds of sitting exercise. Stretch your knees out straight, arch and then bend your lower back, tilt your pelvis, and squeeze in with your abdominal muscles just before standing. You can make this a habit and learn to do it quickly and gracefully so that it does not take thought and is not conspicuous. This little prestanding exercise helps the low back shift gears more smoothly before undergoing major changes in posture.

Once you have done the prestanding exercise, you should position yourself to transfer from sitting to standing with as little low back stress as possible. Put one foot back under the chair a little. Use armrests when they are available, keep your pelvis tilted and your abdomen in, put your weight on the back foot, and then stand straight up and transfer your weight to the front foot.

Riding in Automobiles

Riding in cars or trucks creates special problems for the lower back. You may have to twist to get into and out of cars. The sitting position may be awkward. The tension of driving may be aggravating. The desire to push on may keep you sitting in one position for too long.

If you have a choice of vehicles, it is best to avoid a low-riding, low-sitting sportscar. Higher, roomier cars and trucks are easier to get into and out of and usually permit a better sitting position. An adjustable steering wheel that allows you to slide your knees under the wheel with a minimum of twisting movement is helpful.

Before you get into a car, take a second to check that your back is flat and your pelvis tilted. Be sure that your footing is secure and that the space is clear for you to sit. Don't try to carry anything into the car at the same time as you are getting yourself into it.

Turn backward and sit down in the seat sideways with both feet still on the ground. Use the door and the centerpost of the car as handholds to lower yourself to the seat. Do not throw one leg into the car first and then twist your back as you shift positions and weight at the same time.

Once seated sideways in the seat, legs together and outside the car, allow all your weight to be supported by the seat. Then rotate both legs together with your hips and chest and swing your legs up into the car.

The seat should be adjusted so that your knees are higher than your hips and so that you do not have to reach for the steering wheel. (See Figure 3.) There should be a comfortable, slightly leaning-back position to the backrest. You should not be pushed forward into a directly upright posture. Some of your weight should be taken by the backrest, but if you are driving, you should not have the backrest reclined so far that you have to strain to look forward.

The backrest should give you gentle, firm support across the whole back. The space created by the lumbar lordosis should be filled by the contour of the backrest, but you should not feel as though you are pushed into more lordosis than is natural and comfortable. If the lumbar support of your car's backrest is not adjustable and cannot be made to fit you, you may purchase an adjustable lumbar automobile support from an orthopedic supply shop. A towel roll may serve temporarily.

Your feet should rest comfortably flat on the floor. If your knees must come below hip level to allow you to reach the pedals, you have the seat too far back.

Shoulder seatbelts and neck supports are not only important safety features for the driver and all passengers, but they are also important comfort features. The straps should be snug. You should position the neckrest so that it fits the curve of the neck and allows the back of the skull to rest down on the top of the pad. Your head should not be pushed forward by the neckrest.

If you use your automobile to transport groceries, tools, or other materials, you must take special care when loading and unloading. Don't try to get into the car with packages or even something small, like a purse, in your hands. Set everything down where you want it to be in the car before you get in yourself. Put one foot up on the side of the car (or the bumper if you are loading the trunk) and use proper lifting techniques. Get everything, including children, secure before you get into the car. Don't leave anything unsecure that could tempt you to twist around over the seat to make an adjustment.

If you must take long automobile rides, take a break every hour. Get out, walk around, and do a minute or two of flexibility exercises. Don't sit in one position and drive for hour after hour. That isn't good for your back, and it isn't safe driving. Driving requires a lot of attention—more than experienced drivers realize. Muscle tensions build steadily while driving. You need breaks from that tension as well as from the driving posture.

To get out of a car, you basically reverse the motions of getting in.

Turn both legs at the same time, rotate them with the body to avoid twisting the lower back, make sure that footing and handholds are secure, keep your weight on the seat until you have turned fully and have your feet down, keep one foot a little ahead of the other, tilt the pelvis, and stand. Don't try to lift or carry anything with you as you get out. Wait until you are out, then turn back without twisting and with full attention to good lifting principles, and unload the car.

Lying Down

It is best to lie down on your back or on your side. Stomach sleeping is not recommended, but lying down on the stomach can be done safely and comfortably if a pillow is placed under the hips and lower abdomen.

Most people with back problems are very comfortable lying on their sides. A small pillow between the knees may help. A single pillow that can be flattened down to conform to the head, neck, and shoulder in this position may prevent the neck strain that can be caused by using too many pillows or pillows with too much firmness.

The preferred sleeping position for most people with back pain is on the back with the knees and hips slightly bent. A pillow under the knees is the simplest way to accomplish this.

People who have a lot of leg or sciatic pain may do best with even more bend at the knees and hips. The contour position with the hips and knees bent is similar to the rest position, except that the hips and knees are not bent as much in the contour position. Contoured beds can be purchased, or this bed position may be approximated by putting rolled blankets under the mattress at knee level. Such changes in bed structure are appropriate only for those content to sleep on their backs through the night and, except in the case of an unusually adaptable mate, for those who sleep alone.

You should try to maintain a balanced, neutral lower back posture when sleeping. Pillow props or bed adjustments for the legs are meant to bend the hips and legs, not to give the low back excess flexion. By using only a thin, soft head pillow or no head pillow, you can avoid excess flexion stress to the lower back and to the neck.

Some people need a little support to the lumbar curve while sleeping, similar to that used while sitting. You can tie a rolled towel around your waist to give a little support to the lumbar lordosis and prevent excess flattening while sleeping. If you sleep on your side and experience an uncomfortable sideways sag of the lumbar spine, you may be comfortable if you tie such a roll around your waist to support the down side.

Standard-sized beds may not be comfortable for people much over six feet tall. That may not be a problem until a back condition requires some modification of sleeping posture. Make sure your bed at home is long enough that you don't have to compromise on that account. When you travel, most large hotels and motels will provide extra long beds if you request them in advance.

There is no best orthopedic mattress for people with back pain. Individual preference with consideration to how it feels, durability, appearance, and affordability should be given rather than regarding the mattress as a medically prescribed item. Generally, the mattress should be firm but not rigid. The floor is too hard and a sagging mattress is too soft. A three-quarter-inch plywood board cut to fit under the mattress can firm up an otherwise good one that has become too soft. You can use such a bedboard to vary the hardness from time to time as an experiment to find out what works best for you. Good boxsprings and a reasonably firm mattress usually make bedboards unnecessary, however. Waterbeds are quite satisfactory for some people but uncomfortable for others. The same good sleeping posture principles apply, regardless of the content of the mattress.

After lying down for a long time, particularly after sleeping through the night, take a minute or two to shift gears before standing. Draw your knees up to your chest. Slowly push one leg at a time into full extension at your knees and hips. Tighten your abdomen and tilt your pelvis. Next, turn on one side, draw both knees up, drop your feet over the side of the bed, and push to a sitting position with your arms. Then go through the usual preparation and movements to arise from sitting to standing.

Summary

It doesn't take long to learn correct posture habits, but it may take a while to unlearn any bad habits you may have developed. Your back may have accommodated to some unhealthy postures, so applying the good techniques may seem awkward and uncomfortable. The reward for sticking with it is a more dependable, less painful back. Be especially careful not to lapse back into the old habits when you feel depressed, nervous, angry, or impatient. You will only make bad feelings worse if you aggravate your back condition with improper care.

Applications of these basic principles of standing, sitting, and lying posture will be discussed in the next chapter, which deals with body mechanics and ergonomics—the ways of getting the body to move and perform work properly.

3
BODY MECHANICS

Body mechanics is the study of how we use our bodies to accomplish work. Work in that sense means spending energy to create movement. Work doesn't necessarily mean what we get paid for doing. It certainly doesn't have to mean something unpleasant. It may include all of the things you want to do as well as the things you feel you should do. Included are such activities as taking a walk, lifting a baby, patting a dog, or robbing the refrigerator, as well as the efforts involved in your occupation.

The study of the accomplishment of work is called ergonomics. This includes body mechanics. Ergonomics also includes the study of the design of work equipment and job techniques that are not directly related to body function. Job design and job fitness is discussed in Chapter 10. In this chapter, we will consider the aspects of work that are directly affected by body posture and body movement and are at least partially under your control as you work.

You learned proper methods of standing from Chapter 2. Work that requires standing should be done by following those principles as closely as possible.

It is important to avoid leaning forward with both feet on the floor. Shaving or brushing the teeth while leaning over a low sink are classic examples of poor body mechanics. Bathroom sinks and basins are too low to be used as work surfaces.

Mirrors behind the sink require bending forward for close attention to shaving or makeup. The upper body is forced to rotate in front of the lower back, greatly increasing low back stress. An extensible wall mirror or a hand mirror and avoidance of the habit of unnecessarily close inspection of the face save you from those stresses. A second mirror on a nearby wall also may obviate the need to bend forward over the sink. If you place a stool under the sink and place one foot upon it, you can balance your weight to unload substantially the stresses on your lower back. If there is a cabinet under the sink, you can accomplish the same thing by opening the cabinet door and using the lower shelf to prop one foot.

So, body mechanics can be important from the first acts of your day. Attention to the details of body mechanics while doing such things as brushing your teeth gets you off to a good start by not aggravating the back early in the morning, and it establishes good habits. The same principles that apply to proper tooth brushing apply throughout the day to many tasks you perform while standing.

You may not want to redesign your bathroom sink because it is lower than your ideal work surface, since you spend only a few minutes there each day. If you spend hours each day at the kitchen sink, cooking surface, workbench, or work table, though, the surface height is very important. It should not be so low that you have to lean over or so high that you cannot rest your elbows comfortably upon it. It is ideal if you can vary either the work surface height or your standing surface from time to time. You may be able to use a cutting board to elevate the work surface, an inclined surface so you can vary the height of your attention, or a standing stool so you can raise your standing height. It may also help to sit partially on a high stool some of the time.

Lifting and Bending

Many tasks require the transfer of materials from one surface height to another. Such transfers may involve complex movements that require both lifting and twisting efforts. Proper lifting techniques must be learned first.

The amount of weight that can be lifted safely by an individual depends upon several factors. There are, in fact, so many factors that assigning a limit in terms of pounds has very little meaning unless the other aspects of the task are also defined.

The size, shape, and texture of the object are important variables. How far it must be lifted and from what height, whether it must be carried, and whether twisting and turning are involved are all critical. The number of times the lift must be accomplished, the footing surface characteristics, clothing and other potential hazards, and air temperature may all be important. So, of course, are your individual strengths and abilities at that moment.

There are so many variables in tasks and human capabilities that government and other health agencies have not been able to agree upon regulations to limit lifting. A useful guideline for those willing to delve into the more technical aspects of this problem is *Work Practices Guide for Manual Lifting* from the National Institute of Occupational Safety and Health (NIOSH). It may be obtained for $17.50 by ordering by name and order code PB 82-178-948 from National Technical Information Service, Springfield, Virginia 22161.

Heavy Lifting. Lifting heavy objects from floor level is accomplished most efficiently by using your back for at least some of the lifting effort. (See Figure 4.) If you squat down and bring the object in next to your body, lift it to chest level with your arms, and then rise to standing by lifting with your legs, you can lift rather heavy objects with relatively little

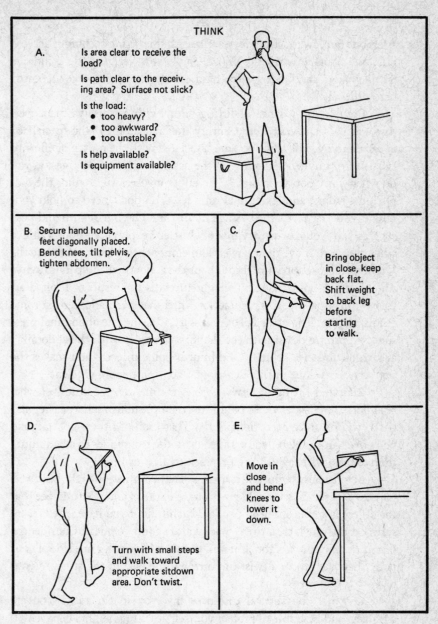

THINK

A. Is area clear to receive the load?

Is path clear to the receiving area? Surface not slick?

Is the load:
- too heavy?
- too awkward?
- too unstable?

Is help available?
Is equipment available?

B. Secure hand holds, feet diagonally placed. Bend knees, tilt pelvis, tighten abdomen.

C. Bring object in close, keep back flat. Shift weight to back leg before starting to walk.

D. Turn with small steps and walk toward appropriate sitdown area. Don't twist.

E. Move in close and bend knees to lower it down.

FIGURE 4. Lifting Heavy Objects.

stress on your lower back. You should learn this lifting technique and use it for occasional heavy lifting. Most people, however, find this technique too inefficient (and perhaps too hard on the knees) to use for repeated heavy lifting.

Precede every stressful lifting effort with a Valsalva maneuver. Antonio Valsalva was a 19th Century Italian anatomist who specialized in ear anatomy. His name became associated with the muscular effort to exhale forcefully while closing off the nasal and oral air passages, as you do when you "pop your ears." The effort involves tightening the diaphragm, trunk, and abdominal muscles. You don't need to hold your nose if you just resist the passage of air through your mouth and nose such as you would when trying to whistle. People often do a Valsalva when trying to move their bowels and empty their bladders because the Valsalva increases pressure throughout the abdominal and pelvic cavity. The grunting noise made by weight lifters is the result of limited air escape during a Valsalva, a practice which has been adopted by some tennis players. The noise is not necessary. Raising the abdominal pressure by pushing down with the diaphragm and in with the abdominal and trunk muscles supports the lumbar spine directly and makes the protective envelope of muscles around the spine more efficient.

Repeated lifting of heavy objects is difficult, regardless of what techniques are mastered. To be able to accomplish such tasks on a regular basis, you must be exceptionally fit. That kind of fitness goes beyond body mechanics. Here, you want to learn the techniques to avoid injury from occasional heavy lifting or repeated lighter lifting.

Before you attempt a lift, make a careful evaluation of the task. Feel for the most secure handhold positions. Be sure of your footing. See that the object is stable and won't suddenly shift after you have lifted it. Be sure that the way is clear to the place you are going to put it. Consider the distribution of the weight. If it will be much heavier for one side of your body than the other, a twisting force will be part of the stress to your back.

Consider the vertical distances involved in the task. You are strongest and best able to protect yourself at lifting heights between 30 and 50 inches from the floor. Lifting from floor level is much more difficult than lifting from 12 or more inches above your standing surface. It is also much more difficult to lift higher than chest level.

Before you commit yourself to the lift, test the weight to make sure you can manage it. If you are not sure you can handle it, get help. Even if you think you can manage it, if equipment or help is available, use them. If the load can be divided, take two or more trips.

When you squat, either fully or partially, and pull an object in close to your body, it is best to have one foot in front of the other. You balance the forces best if you use the hand opposite the forward foot as the lead hand. This creates a diagonal direction of force, minimizing the stress created by twisting the lower back. This is a comfortable and effective way to deal with lifting, pushing, and pulling. Once you learn it, it is easy to make it a habit.

It is important to keep the weight of the object in close to your body. (See Figure 5.) Experiments have been performed in which instruments that measure the stress on lumbar discs have been inserted into the spines of volunteers. The results show that the greatest stresses are caused by efforts to lift objects that are away from the body.

It is also known from experiments that the ligaments that are most important for holding the discs in place, those of the anulus fibrosus, are most vulnerable when twisting forces are applied. The fibers of these ligaments take a short oblique course from the body of one vertebra to the next. It takes a tremendous force to rupture those fibers by pulling straight out on them. Like the force it takes to tear a phone book in two, a strong twisting force may isolate and tear individual fibers until the ligament ruptures.

The two most important things to remember when attempting a heavy lift are to get the weight in close to your body and to avoid twisting. Whenever possible, you should gain full control of the weight, stand, turn, and then set it down. Don't try to rotate from one position to the other by twisting your body. You don't have to take a lot of extra steps to avoid twisting. Pivot on the heel of the foot nearest your destination, just as a soldier would when doing a "right face" or "left face."

Some activities, such as prolonged shoveling, can be accomplished

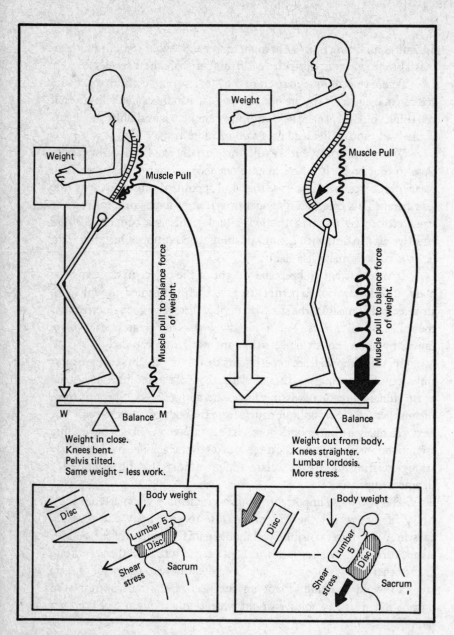

FIGURE 5. Mechanics of Lifting.

efficiently only by twisting with heavy loads. Such activities can be done for long periods only by exceptionally fit people. Those less fit may learn to do such things for shorter periods of time and with a compromise of the work efficiency.

Don't lift weights that are clearly beyond what you are accustomed to doing. Except in rare emergencies, it is not worth the risk of back injury. Two people can lift much more safely than one. Repeated very heavy lifting should be done with equipment.

Intermediate Lifting. Many people who have had back trouble can work regularly at jobs or can return to activities that require a moderate amount of lifting. To do so safely, they must learn and practice proper techniques and be careful to keep themselves fit for the tasks.

Some tasks require bending to beyond 45 degrees and do not allow you to squat or kneel. You may have to reach over something and lift a moderately heavy object from the floor. When you do, you should keep your lower back stiff and straight. Your hips will allow you to bend without bending your lower back. This technique will seem unnatural at first because you must contract your back muscles much more forcefully than you would if you allowed your back to bend. The extra effort is well worth the protection it provides to the ligaments and discs of your back. Practice this technique by bending forward with a yardstick laying along the midline of your back. Keep the entire stick in contact with your back as you bend.

If you keep your back muscles strong, it doesn't hurt them to do some lifting, especially in the range from upright to 45 degrees. It isn't necessary to keep your back rigidly upright to protect your back muscles. Once you exceed 45 degrees of forward bending, you place more stress on the structures of the lower back and demand more of the back muscles. When the task requires bending over that far, it becomes much more important to use the techniques for heavy lifting.

The muscles of the buttocks, the hip extensors and abductors, can become quite strong if they are exercised. They can bear much of the brunt of heavy lifting. One reason why it is important to bend the hips and knees when lifting is that these muscles are in the position to function with greatest strength when the hips are flexed. Also, by bending the hips and knees, you get the object in closer to your body and thereby decrease the leverage of the weight against your lower back. Control of the knees and power to lift the weight by straightening the knees depend upon strong thigh muscles.

Lifting children presents special, usually pleasurable, lifting problems. The needs for special security and provision for sudden movements are balanced by the child's ability to assist with the task. You best protect your back if you drop to one knee, allow time in that position for you and the child to adjust securely to one another, and then rise.

If you learn proper techniques of lifting with special emphasis on keeping the weight in close, avoid excessive bending and twisting, and control the knees and hips with strong thigh and buttock muscles, you can do a considerable amount of lifting without harm to your back.

Light Lifting. When you bend over to lift a very light object, the problem is with the bend rather than the lift. You should put all of your weight on your forward leg. Steady one arm either by holding on to the forward knee as you bend it or by holding on to any available knee-high object. As you grasp the object with your free hand, lift your rear leg off the floor and use it as a counterbalance.

Balance is the most important part of light lifting. If your effort will be uncoordinated because your back hurts or the surface is slippery, do not hesitate to squat or kneel even if it is just to lift a handkerchief.

Setting Objects Down. When you lift, hold, and set down objects, avoid standing with both feet flat together. Keep one foot forward. When standing still or preparing to walk with an object, have most of the weight on the back foot.

As you prepare to set an object down, place your forward foot as close to the height of the surface as practical so that you avoid leaning forward with the weight. For example, when you set a grocery bag down into an automobile trunk, put your forward foot or your knee on the bumper. That will diminish the stress on your back as you lower the bag into the trunk. When possible, get your forward knee under the surface as when setting an object on a table with a clear space under it.

Pushing and Pulling

Much of the focus on the causes of back pain is on lifting. Pushing and pulling also produce back stress. The essential features of safe pushing and pulling are the same as those of lifting. Keep control of the situation, do not try to do what is beyond what you are accustomed to doing, keep one foot in front of the other, use the diagonal principle to balance your body and the force you are exerting, keep close to the object, and keep your hips and knees bent.

When you evaluate a task which involves pushing or pulling efforts, it is most important to consider the surfaces. The friction and stability of the standing surface limit the force you can exert through your feet. The friction and inclination of the contact points between the object and the surface it is to slide or roll upon determine the forces needed to move it. It is safer for your back if the object is to be pushed straight than if it must be guided to one side.

It requires more force to start, stop, or change direction than it does to sustain motion. You must evaluate what will be required to stop the object once it begins moving. More injuries occur because of inability to stop a pushed object safely than because of the pushing effort that kept it going.

When you have a choice of either pushing or pulling a heavy object, it is usually easier on your back to push it. Make the contact of your hands with the object somewhere around shoulder level. Make as much body contact as you can with the object. It is especially helpful to get your forward leg against it and push directly with that leg. Avoid twisting.

Some people can push things with more ease than they can do almost anything else. They find that leaning forward a little and pushing, such as when pushing a grocery cart, relieves back and leg discomfort. This is particularly true of people with spinal stenosis, a back condition in which pinched nerves are sometimes relieved by leaning forward.

Reaching

Lifting heavy objects above chest level can be very stressful to the lower back and should be avoided by those who are not conditioned to do so. Reaching up and lifting an object off a high shelf may be especially dangerous. (See Figure 6.) It is best to use a stepladder or a standing platform. Be sure the object is something you can handle. Do all you can to prepare for it before you get compromised with it in hand in an awkward position.

Frequent lifting of light to moderate objects from high shelves is a common problem for store clerks, librarians, and homemakers. Small stepladders and standing stools with casters can save a lot of back stress. When reaching up it is important to do a pelvic tilt and when you make the lifting effort to do a Valsalva.

When you are having back trouble, you should avoid tasks that require prolonged effort above chest level. If work must be done high up, use a stepladder or a raised platform. If you cannot elevate yourself to a position of comfort for a particular task, such as painting a ceiling, do the job in short sessions.

Some tasks require you to reach forward and pull objects toward you at or above waist level. If you need to make such efforts frequently, you may have less back pain if you use a cane or crook to catch and pull the objects in closer to you.

Sitting Work and Work Furniture

The chair and desk become integral parts of the body mechanics for people who do most of their work while sitting. Sitting posture habits (as discussed in Chapter 2) are especially important for people who sit while

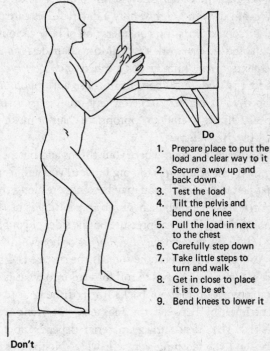

Do

1. Prepare place to put the load and clear way to it
2. Secure a way up and back down
3. Test the load
4. Tilt the pelvis and bend one knee
5. Pull the load in next to the chest
6. Carefully step down
7. Take little steps to turn and walk
8. Get in close to place it is to be set
9. Bend knees to lower it

Don't

1. Take on loads of unknown size, weight, or distribution
2. Lift down from above head
3. Let back sway in as weight comes down
4. Let neck extend as weight is held
5. Twist to set the load down

FIGURE 6. Lifting Down from a Height.

working. So are flexibility and relaxation exercises. In this section, however, the emphasis will be on work furniture.

Most people are accustomed to selection of chairs for their homes based upon appearance and short-term comfort. Selection of a chair in which you are to spend eight hours a day requires care and knowledge about chair components and consideration of how various chair features can be adapted to the work tasks. Most chair designs are based upon measurements of the human body called *anthropomorphics*. Most chair features fit the middle 80 percent of those anthropomorphic measurements, so if you are a very large or very small person you may need to make special efforts to find an appropriate chair or make special adaptations of what is available.

The surface of a chair where your thighs and buttocks rest is called the *seat pan*. If the seat pan is too big for you, you will feel unsupported. If the seat pan is too small, you may become sore along the sides of your hips. A little less than two inches of foam padding is usually best. If the pad is too thick it will create pressure on the sides of your hips and if it is too thin it will cause the *ischial tuberosities,* or boney knobs of the pelvis under your buttocks, to become sore. If the surface is dished out at the back it will allow your pelvis to roll forward into what is usually a more comfortable position for your back. If it is dished out under each thigh with a little ridge between the legs near the front it may be more comfortable. The ideal surface material depends upon temperature, humidity, and the clothing you will wear. Nonporous materials may become too hot, and slick materials may cause you to slide around too easily, especially if you wear clothing with a low friction surface.

The seat pan is usually parallel to the floor. If the task calls for it, such as frequent needs to lean and reach forward, it may be best that the seat pan incline forward about five degrees. Some chairs feature seat pans which can be adjusted to be inclined forward, flat, or leaned back to about ten degrees. Some feature automatic adjustments so that the seat pan inclination will vary in response to forces placed upon it.

The seat pan fit affects and is affected by the backrest. Some chairs have seat pans which can be adjusted forward and backward in relation to the backrest. Most work chairs have backrests which are at least partially adjustable as to height and inclination.

The chair-fit characteristic which is most important to the support of your lower back is the lumbar support. The height of the backrest relative to the seat pan should be such that the lumbar support of the backrest contacts you at about the belt line. Backrests should not contact your shoulder blades except when leaning back in executive style chairs. There should be firm support of the lumbar lordosis over a wide area of your lower back. Adjustments of seat pan and backrest positions should focus on the need for good lumbar support. Once the lumbar support is fitted to the correct place, the pressure of it may be adjusted either by a tension spring or by adjusting the inclination of the backrest and the position of the seat pan.

The distance from the floor to the seat pan is adjustable in most work chairs. Simple manual height adjustment mechanisms are adequate for most chairs. Pneumatic pushbutton or lever adjustments are easier though more expensive. If frequent changes of the height of the chair help relieve back fatigue or are necessary to your particular job, the pneumatic feature may be worth the investment.

The proper height of the chair depends upon the height of the work surface. You can elevate your legs by using a footrest, so it is of primary importance to adjust the height of the seat pan so that your upper body is properly positioned. For more desk work you will want your elbows to be at or about an inch below the table height. Unless you are very tall or very short or work at an unusual height, you will find most chairs are made to be adjustable in that range. Stools with most of the other features discussed here are available for those who work at higher than usual surfaces. Many such stools are height adjustable over a greater range than are most chairs.

If you work with your hands at one level through much of the day, you may find it better to have some support for your forearms. Armrests on your chair may provide that. Armrests also make getting into and out of the chair easier when your back is hurting. Armrests may get in the way if your work requires moving from one station to another, so either try it both ways before you decide or use a chair with easily detachable armrests. It is important that the armrests are low and recessed enough that they do not strike the desk or prevent you from getting close to your work surface.

You want to keep both feet comfortably flat so your hips are bent to right angles and the weight of your legs is taken by the floor. If your legs are short and your work surface high, you may need foot support. A simple wood block of the proper height may be adequate if you do not move around much. An inclined wood block allows you to vary the height of your legs and the angles of your knees and hips. Even if you have no problem placing your feet flat on the floor, you may find that using a footstool or inclined board for one or both feet helps dispel fatigue and backache. Most stools and many chairs have a circular rim around the pedestal or a stirrup suspended from the seat pan which can be used as foot rests.

Most work chairs are supported by a single pedestal. The stability of the chair depends upon blades which radiate from the base of the pedestal. The length and number of the blades are determinants of the stability. Most chairs have either four or five blades, the latter being more stable. Your need for stability is greater if you work with the chair adjusted high, if you move around and in and out of the chair frequently, and if you lean in the chair.

Most work chairs make contact with the floor through casters. Casters should allow you to move about easily in your chair, so that minor adjustments in the distance from your work can be made to suit your comfort and so that you can move from one work station to another without leaning and twisting your back. They should not move so easily that the chair moves with every shift of your body weight. If the chair moves too easily, you will feel unsteady in it and the chair will feel unstable to you when you sit down into it or arise from it. The function of the casters depends on their design and the type of surface they will contact. Casters are made for either a hard surface or for carpet. Hard surface casters will not function properly on carpet and carpet casters are not safe on hard surfaces. Most casters are easy to change so you don't need to limit your chair selection by this feature. Some jobs are done better in chairs without casters, in which case you can have the casters replaced with glides.

Most work chairs follow the basic design described above. One innovative variation is the kneeling chair. It has no backrest. The seat pan inclines forward. Your knees rest on a padded board. The lumbar lordosis is maintained by body position rather than a lumbar support. It is particularly suitable for working over a low flat surface.

There has been a great deal of research and progress in work chair design in recent years, mostly because of the problem of back pain. As a result there are many excellent chairs available which incorporate some or all of the above features. The limiting factor is cost. Chairs which are well made and incorporate many features for back support are expensive. They are not as expensive as back pain, but they are expensive enough that you should consider carefully what you need and try out several models before you make a purchase.

You may not need a new chair at all. Most of the features described have been available on work chairs for a long time. They are too often ignored. People inherit a chair with a job and never make the proper adjustments. Lumbar supports are improperly placed and tension never adjusted. Tension springs and adjustment mechanisms go without simple maintenance. Seat pan heights are left at the height proper to the previous occupant who may have been several inches taller or shorter. Casters wear out and don't work properly or a carpet is installed or a carpet-saver surface placed under the chair and appropriate changes in the casters never made. Chair maintenance and chair adjustments are simple and inexpensive. If everyone gave attention to those details it would obviate the need for a lot of expensive new chair purchases and a lot of back care.

For most situations it is easier to change the chair than to change the work surface. Adjustment of the work surface height is an alternative to some of the alterations which can be made on work chairs. This is particularly true of work which is done standing or on a high stool. Standing work surface height is usually best when your elbows are about two inches above the surface. Desks and work tables must have enough clearance under them so that you can move yourself and your chair next to the work surface without compromising your leg comfort or leaning away from the backrest.

Computers have radically changed the nature of sitting work for many people. The keyboard and video display terminal have, for thousands of workers, replaced the typewriter and file cabinets. The result is that the work station has become smaller and the opportunity to move around during the course of work has diminished. Fatigue and tension may be greater among video display operators because of the confined attention to one area. The rapid expansion of computer use in homes and schools makes attention to details of work station design and proper chairs important to homemakers and students as well as workers.

Design for ease of vision is particularly important for video display terminal operators. The distance of the screen from your eyes should be between 17½ and 20 inches. The angle between your eyes and the center of the screen should be 10 to 20 degrees. The top of the screen should not be above eye level and the bottom not below 40 degrees downward. Lighting requires special attention because the light necessary for easy reading of hard copy might interfere with ease of reading from the screen. Provisions must be made to have the hard copy material at a comfortable level and lighted adequately.

Computer keyboard height recommendations are similar to those for typewriters. With your fingers at the home position on the keyboard your elbows should be bent between 80 and 120 degrees and your elbows should be at or slightly below table height. That means, for most people, the home row of the keyboard should be 28 to 31 inches above the floor. Distance from the floor, however, is not the important variable if proper adjustments of chair height, desk clearance, and foot support are made. Some video display terminals have movable keyboards which may allow you to vary the height of the keyboard quite easily if you can still maintain the requirements for adequate vision of the screen.

Little League Parent Syndrome

Not all backaches from sitting are related to the work place. The worst possible circumstances for sitting befall parents who sit for hours watching their children perform athletics. Bleacher seats are often crowded and make squirming for comfort difficult. The sitting surface can hardly be called a seat pan. There is no lumbar support. There are no armrests and no footrests. Nothing is adjustable. The duration of events may be quite long. Anxieties may run high and if your child's team is losing you may not get many chances to stand up and relieve your tension.

If you spend many hours as a sports fan it is well worth it to your back to purchase a good portable stadium seat. It will at least give you some seat padding and a little lumbar support. Try to sit on the edge of the bleachers or near the aisle where it will be easier for you to get up periodically. Take every opportunity to cheer and when you do, stand up and extend your back. Don't let your children's exercise be your vicarious participation in athletics. You need exercise and recreation in which you are an active participant.

Scheduling Work

If the requirements of your job allow it, it is best to do demanding tasks in short segments. It is common for people to hurt their backs by working all day in a spring garden, doing something they have not done for months. Similar injuries occur from many sports and work activities. Often, the activities could have been done without injury if the duration of effort had been shorter on the first few attempts.

A new task or a task that has not been done in a long time should be approached with some caution. The same stress that causes strong calluses on the hands if done in short segments over several days will produce painful blisters and leave tender hands if done all at one time. The same is true of backs. Spring gardeners, weekend athletes, and occasional laborers, take heed.

4
DAILY HABITS

You must be concerned with the preservation of your health throughout 24 hours of every day. Your body is not like an automobile that can be replaced if you damage it. Even the few artificial body parts that medical technology makes available are not wholly satisfactory. The lower back does not contain any parts that have been replaced with even partial success, so maintenance of the one you have is your only choice.

Back pain may just be one, perhaps the first, symptom of inadequate health maintenance. If you respond by improving your attitude toward the care of your health, the back pain could turn out to be a fortunate occurrence. The steps you take to treat your back pain may result in improved general health and may prevent a more costly and less reparable breakdown. The important daily habits of proper nutrition and exercise will be discussed in Chapters 7 and 12.

The ideal duration of sleep is an individual thing, but many people feel uncertain about what is right for them. Chronic lack of sleep from overwork or worry certainly is unhealthy and may aggravate the problems that cause back pain. On the other hand, many people who are prone to stiffness and aching muscles and joints have more trouble if they sleep for too long at a time.

Most healthy people sleep about seven hours each day. Some people seem to need a little more or a little less. People who do general fitness exercises on a regular basis usually require less sleep than others. Duration of sleep is partially related to habit.

Sleep should be restorative. Once you are fully awake, you should feel fresh and ready to start again. Achieving the feeling of being restored is more important than the number of hours you slept. Sleeping periods that are too long or too short may be factors in nonrestorative sleeping, but they are not the only factors.

Sleeping pills frequently do not result in restorative sleep. Many people wake up too soon when they have taken sleeping pills, or they wake up feeling hung over. In certain instances when some situation makes falling asleep the only sleep problem, a sleeping pill may be helpful, but more often they do more harm than good. Nonrestorative sleeping and trouble sleeping through the night because of depression sometimes may be relieved by antidepressant prescription drugs.

Alcohol may be a major part of some people's sleeping problems. If you drink late in the evening, the alcohol is likely to make you sleepy. Too often, the result is that you fall asleep only to awaken before you have been restored by sleep.

Sleeping medication or alcohol may be the whole problem. Quitting both results in normal sleep for some people. There may be a delay time while the body adjusts to the withdrawal of these drugs, and during that time it may be harder to fall asleep.

Medicine is seldom a complete answer to a sleeping problem. Selection of the proper drug and dosage may be difficult. Don't experiment with someone else's sleeping medicine or over-the-counter drugs. Consult your doctor if you think drugs have to be part of the solution.

Be aware that sleeping problems are not isolated problems. They are usually symptoms of other things that are wrong. Inadequate exercise, excessive medication or alcohol, and unresolved emotional conflicts are the most common complications.

Back pain is usually relieved by rest in the proper position. If your back pain has become acutely worse, it may make it more difficult to sleep at first. If you know the proper sleeping postures and relaxation techniques, you should be able to overcome that problem before long. The common forms of back pain seldom result in prolonged difficulty with sleeping. If you are consistently awakened in the middle of the night by back pain and have more pain through the night than at other times, you should consult further with your doctor to be sure that you do not have some unusual problem.

Getting Up

No matter how long or how short your sleeping period, awaken yourself with ample time to go through your routine at a relaxed pace. A common characteristic of people who live with too much tension and unnecessary stress is that when they get up in the morning they are already a little behind. They leave no time margin to accommodate any extra problem or pleasure.

There are also physical reasons to allow yourself extra time in the mornings. The intervertebral discs, which are the source of difficulty for many people, are a little swollen in the early morning. Their center imbibes water when you are off your feet. The longer the recumbency period, the more swollen they may be. Ligaments and muscles shorten a little at complete rest and also may be sources of early morning pain. Therefore, if you have slept long, you need to take extra time to avoid excessive stress to the lower back shortly after arising. If you are going to a physically stressful job in the morning or plan some early morning athletic activity, it is especially important to get up early enough to allow your back to adjust.

Calculate the time it takes to do all of the things you need to do in the morning before your first commitment. Figure in ample time for exercise, bathing, eating at a normal pace, and relaxed driving. Total up the time and then give yourself 10 to 15 extra minutes. If something goes wrong or something extra comes up, you have plenty of time for it. If everything goes according to schedule, you have a bonus of extra time for your pleasure or to be early for your first scheduled activity. If you start off your day a little ahead instead of a little behind, you have a hedge against stress that is worth much more than the 10 to 15 minutes of sleep you gave up for it.

Clothing

Freedom of motion, especially around the hips, is very important for normal back function and prevention of back injury. Flexibility exercises restore and preserve such motion. It does little good to have free joint motion, however, if tight fitting clothing restricts ease of movement. It is especially important to allow free motion of the hips and knees when performing physical work or doing exercises. Avoid clothing which binds you through the groin or at the bends of the knees or that pinches your waist as you bend forward.

When working or exercising in cold weather it is important to stay warm without restricting motion or creating hazards. Bulky coats and jackets restrict motion, add extra weight to the stress on your lower back, and present the threat of catching in something. Hats provide extra warmth without those disadvantages. Wearing properly-fitting long underwear, long socks, and warm pants may allow you to stay warm without overloading your upper body.

A wide belt which can be cinched tightly about the waist may act as a first aid and preventive device during heavy work. Weightlifters have long used such belts. An elastic abdominal binder worn under the shirt may provide similar support and additional warmth to a sore back.

Shoe wear is very important. Select sole characteristics which allow you to accomplish the task with the least chance of slipping. The friction provided by good rubber soles with waffle or other high friction design are safest for pushing, pulling, jogging, hiking, and many other activities. Shoes with a wide heel and well-fitting heel counters provide additional stability. High-heeled shoes tend to throw your body forward, forcing you to push your back into excess lordosis to maintain balance. High heels also increase the threat of injury from falling. If you must wear high-heeled shoes, try to avoid standing for long in one place, stay on flat, stable surfaces, and hold onto rails or someone's arm whenever possible.

Smoking

Once you are off to such a good start, you want to continue throughout your day to do things that are in the best interest of your health. One of the most common things that many people do to the detriment of their health is to smoke.

Nothing that modern people commonly do voluntarily is as devastating to health as smoking. The testimonials, circumstantial evidence, and statistical evidence that document the harms of smoking are overwhelming.

It may seem, at first, a little bit off the point to make strong statements about the harmful effects of smoking in a book about back care. Smoking is, after all, well known as a cause of damage to the heart, lungs, and blood vessels, but not to the spine.

Actually, it has been shown statistically that people who smoke are more likely to rupture lumbar discs. It has not been shown clearly what the causal relationship is or even if there is one. It may be that the damage smoking does to blood vessels interferes with the already precarious circulation of the discs. It may be that coughing from smoke-induced lung damage exerts excessive stress on the discs. It may be that people who care little enough about their health to smoke ignore other important aspects of health maintenance.

More important than any statistical or theoretical links between smoking and disc ruptures are the effects of smoking on the quality of life. The common disorders that cause back pain are not a threat to life itself. The pain they produce diminishes the quality of life. The effort to triumph over back pain is an effort to improve the quality of life. If you are seriously compromising the quality of your life in other ways, such as by smoking, it makes it more difficult to take steps to overcome your back pain.

Smoking seriously impairs the functions of lungs, heart, and blood vessels. It doesn't just occasionally cause loss of life from lung cancer or heart attack for some few unlucky people. It impairs everyone. Your health, the quality of your life, and your ability to conquer other problems, like back pain, will be improved if you do not smoke.

Healthy Days

Make good health practices a routine part of your entire day. Pay attention to your posture and use good body mechanics. Set aside time for regular exercise and do relaxation, posture, and stretching exercises throughout the day. Observe the rules of good nutrition. Keep the attitude that you are in charge of your health, that you are not going to allow yourself to do things that will be detrimental to your health, and that you are not going to allow unnecessary interference with your pursuit of a healthy mind and body.

5
PSYCHOLOGICAL FACTORS

No one seems surprised when headaches are said to be caused by fatigue, anger, frustration, or nervousness. The relationship between psychological tension and back pain has not received as much media coverage as has that between emotion and headache or upset stomach. The public is not as quick to associate back pain with frustration. Those who care for many people who suffer with back pain certainly see the relationship, and those who have suffered from back pain for long often come to see how psychological factors aggravate their back pains, if they do not bring them on. Everyone recognizes that psychological tensions can result in fatigue and muscle tension. It is not a big step from that recognition to identifying at least one link between emotional stress and back pain.

Sometimes, the psychological aspect of a back pain problem is the most important factor. At other times, it may not be the initiating factor or the major factor, but it always plays some role. Even under conditions, such as elective surgery, where the amount of physical disturbance is predictable, the pain response of any given individual may vary a great deal depending upon psychological factors. Anxiety and depression always make back pain worse, regardless of the origin of the pain.

Do You Think It's All in My Head?

You may worry that someone, perhaps your boss or your doctor, thinks your pain is all in your head. You may have wondered if such a thing might be true about yourself. The very nature of the question reveals a misunderstanding about pain.

Pain is not something that is "out there." There is no such substance as pain. Pain can't be measured in a test tube, poured on or stuck in from the outside, or cut out by a surgeon's blade.

Throughout your body, there are nerve endings that may be stimulated in various ways by different substances or events. Stimulation of the nerve endings initiates a message that is relayed along nerves, through nerve cells, and across nerve connections until it reaches the part of your brain that interprets the message to produce a conscious thought about the event.

Whether that message ever arrives and actually stimulates conscious awareness depends upon how many similar messages are sent at the same time, how well those messages cross the nerve connections and travel along the nerves, and how responsive the nerve cells are to those messages. Whether the messages, once received, are interpreted as pain depends upon all of those factors and upon your mind's interpretation of what the signal means.

The experience of pain, therefore, is something much more complex than simply identification of the stimulus. Pain is not always something bad. In fact, it is usually a helpful warning that you are doing something wrong, something that could be harmful to your body.

You can think of pain as an alarm system, such as the smoke alarm system meant to protect a building from destruction by fire. If a fire occurs, the alarm goes off, and an effort is made to put out the fire. That is how it should work. If a smoke alarm system is too sensitive, every bit of dust or cigarette smoke might set off the alarm. The repeated and unnecessary responses to the alarm could become damaging.

Some people have pain alarm systems that are too sensitive. Some people are just born that way, some have their pain sensitivity heightened by psychological or unrelated physical factors, and some people seem to develop increased sensitivity after they have suffered pain for a long time. Too many pain messages get through, and messages about stimuli that ordinarily would be harmless get interpreted as being from harmful, painful stimuli.

Your body has natural protective mechanisms that keep the system from being too sensitive. You can impair this natural protection if you take pain-relieving and tranquilizing drugs or if you do not get enough exercise. This partially explains why such drugs fail to relieve chronic pain, why pain increases when such drugs are withdrawn, and why exercise helps to relieve chronic pain.

The pain recognition system may be too sensitive if your mind is troubled by other problems that are causing anxiety or depression. Some people become conditioned by their life circumstances to be overly responsive to pain stimuli or to misinterpret ordinarily tolerable stimuli as something harmful.

Your mind is usually occupied by many different events, sensations, and thoughts. All of these things can be interpreted in many different ways, and varying degrees of importance may be assigned to each. The context in which your mind receives stimuli that could be interpreted as painful can be varied by changes in life circumstances and by willful alterations of your mental outlook. Simple examples are the lack of awareness of otherwise very painful injuries by athletes during competition or soldiers in battle.

The question, "Is it all in my mind?" must always be answered, "Yes." This does not mean that the pain is made up in a simple, conscious way. All pains, even those from obvious external causes such as cuts or burns, are in the mind. Only the stimuli that affect the nerve endings are "out there." The pain that is in the mind depends on those stimuli, all the nerve hookups and relays, and the attitude of the mind when the message reaches the part of the brain that brings the event to consciousness.

Backs and Life During Middle Age

Physical changes that can cause back pain occur in the lower back during middle age, the thirties, forties, and fifties. Common mechanical back pain and pain related to disc disorders are much less common among children, adolescents, and older people. These middle years, when changes that may cause pain are occurring in the anatomy of the back, are for most people years of great psychological stress.

Housewives are burdened with the care of children. They suffer through the problems of school and adolescence with their children, and then they face the void that is left in their lives as the kids leave home.

Work that may have held promise and challenge at first may have become boring because of repetition. The physical demands of work that seemed easy in one's twenties become less tolerable as the strength and resilience of youth fade.

Difficult choices of compromise to the demands of family, financial obligations, and career become more frequent. Alternatives diminish.

Age and specialization of skills may make for fewer possibilities to change jobs or locations. This may lead to needs to compromise with the demands of the present job. The company, the boss, or the coworkers may be unpleasant to work with but impossible to avoid without leaving the security of the job.

Marriages may fail or hang together with tension and strife. Parents age and can become burdensome where they once were supportive. Friends suffer illnesses or failures or move away.

All of these stresses are much more common in one's thirties, forties, or fifties than they were in one's twenties. The middle years are the ones in which people must face the frustrations of lost hopes and dreams yet must go on supporting themselves, their children, and perhaps their parents.

These are also the years when backs start to fail. It is no wonder that there is a strong interrelationship between back pain and anxiety and depression.

Back Pain As an Escape

For some people, back pain can become a means of escape. If it all seems too much and they feel overwhelmed, the first thing to go may be back function. Being down with back pain may mean an escape from a job that seems overwhelming. It may mean that the spouse and kids have to demand less. It may mean that less guilt is felt for not being able to keep up with it all.

Back Pain As an Expression of Anger

Sometimes when it seems there is no other way to express anger, some people will express it through back pain. If a worker is hurt doing a job he or she should not have had to do, or doing a job he or she feels is beneath his or her abilities, or serving an overly demanding and unappreciative boss, the anger and frustration is sometimes expressed as back pain.

It always seems to hurt more and longer if we are injured doing something we didn't want to do, particularly if it was someone else's idea that we do it. Teenagers who suffer all sorts of blows without a complaint while on the athletic field may be very vocal in their suffering if they bump themselves doing a chore at home. Husbands and wives may be sick or in pain, therefore unable to do something for the other, when the real reason why they don't want to do it is that they are angry about something else.

Pushing Through Pain to More Pain

Some people react to back pain in a way that seems designed to cause more back pain. They may not be angry with anyone or trying to escape anything. They may have nothing at all to gain from being down with back pain. These people, usually hard-driving, type A personalities, react to pain as though it angers them, and they refuse to care for themselves properly when pain occurs. These people, who often live and function in spite of a great deal of stress, accept the pain as one more stress and just push that much harder. The back pain adds one more source of tension to an already overstressed life. The back pain makes their tension worse, and the tension makes their back pain worse. The cycle must lead eventually either to breakdown or to a change in behavior with self-recognition of the need for proper care.

Fear of Back Pain

Fear of pain is one of the major obstacles to recovery from a back condition. People who have had painful experiences with their backs are often afraid to try anything that might risk return of the pain. Those who have made some kind of adjustment to living with a back problem, no matter how unsuccessful, may be unwilling to try methods that would lead to greater success, because they are afraid to lose the balance they have gained.

Most people who have given up work because of back pain really want to go back to work but are afraid to do so because of fear of back pain or fear of not being able to adjust to the job situation. Most people who have given up family responsibilities, sex, or recreation would like to return to full function and would do so were it not for fear of the consequences. Fear that things could get worse stands in the way of any attempt to make things better.

The major theme of this book is that the risks you take to recover from back pain are worth it. The price you pay if you don't take them is too high. If you are armed with the right tools, the odds that you will get better are overwhelmingly in your favor. If you use the methods you learn in this book, your chances of success are so great that you will overcome the fears and take the risks of doing things that lead to wellness.

People who get some help or compensation and are relieved from the stresses of their lives because of back pain often do so at great expense. While the middle years are ones of considerable stress, they are also ones of great productivity and joy.

The frustrations of raising children are coupled with the joys. The more one participates in it, the greater the reward, both at the time and later. Most people have developed skills and maturity in their work and can call upon experience or seniority in their jobs to gain more favorable circumstances. Most jobs are done better and faster by people with some experience. The satisfactions derived from doing a job well should be greatest for most people in their middle years. Friendships and love relationships should be more mature and giving than those of youth.

People who drop out of the stresses of middle life because of back pain also drop out of full appreciation of the rewards. The long-range cost of this dropout is often much greater than it may seem at first. Some of the social implications of this are discussed in more detail in Chapter 11. Here we will consider primarily the psychological effects.

Regular, productive work, whether from an outside public job or home-based self-employment such as homemaking or farming, is necessary for the psychological health of most people. Too much of what we all see and know of as life is lost if we are not productive. Even if absence from work seems to be well tolerated at first, it seldom is so in the long run. Most people who do not work become depressed or develop behavior patterns that destroy their relationships with others and rob them of the joy in their lives.

Gains obtained by absences from work, withdrawal from home responsibility, or avoiding obligations in personal relationships may seem very nice at first. Back pain as a mechanism to make those gains may seem very easy. However, a habit pattern can develop. Less and less pain may be used to gain more and more escape. The effect can be almost like using drugs or alcohol to escape from problems. What seems harmless enough at first can become very destructive.

The use of drugs and alcohol is a particularly meaningful comparison for reasons beyond demonstration of how addictions and dependency develop. Sometimes drugs, medicines, or alcohol can become the primary problem. To justify taking more pills or another drink, you must have more pain. The confusion between the need for drugs or a drink and back pain may become great enough that the pain comes in response to the need for alcohol or medicine.

The link between back pain and escape from stress leads to the development of behavior patterns. Employers, coworkers, family, and friends who were very glad to be helpful at first become less tolerant of compromises they have to make because of another's pain. This means that to go on getting those rewards the pain must be exaggerated more and more. This exaggeration may be made not only to those directly involved but also to doctors, leading to more and more tests and treatments.

Very few people ever enter this sort of cycle intentionally. No one who sees the full picture of it and the end result ever would. No amount of escape from problems or financial or other reward is worth what this does to people.

People get into these habits barely aware or sometimes totally unaware of what they are doing. They may get encouraged in it by well-meaning friends, spouses, union advisors, attorneys, or medical practitioners. Very few people ever get into this cycle because it is all in their heads. Almost all really do have something wrong with their backs. Frequently, the problem with the anatomy of the back is a very serious one, which really does require some treatment or compromise of function. The problem is that, as people get caught in this spiral, the treatments and the compromises can become much more devastating than the disease.

Recognition of Psychological Factors

The first step toward relieving the harmful psychological aspects of back pain is to recognize them. Many times, just taking an honest look at the possibilities will lead to such a recognition. It may be difficult to look objectively at these possibilities. People fear the inference that the pain is all in the head or that they have mental problems. Both of these inferences are inaccurate oversimplifications of the problem and should not be allowed to prevent an honest look at the situation.

Keeping a diary may help you to see some of the relationships between psychological factors and back pain. Detailed logging of back pain symptoms may be too time-consuming to do for a long period, but important information often can be gleaned from two or three weeks of careful diary keeping. The diary should include all of the times you experience back pain. The intensity and duration of the pains should be noted. Placing the intensity on a scale from one to ten may simplify it.

Besides a chronicle of your back pain, the diary should be a careful, honest log of all of the things that bother you. Be picky and include every little thing, even things that don't seem to matter very much. The cumulative effects of repeated little irritations that you dismiss because you think they shouldn't bother you may add up to major annoyance and tension. The value of the diary is that you can see the effects of these things and their correlation with back pain over a period of several days or weeks. You may recognize patterns that were not apparent when you faced the stresses of life one by one and hour by hour.

Planning Psychological Self-Help

You need to have honest talks with the people to whom you are closest. You need to know from your spouse, your kids, your boss, your coworkers, and your friends where you really stand with them. You need to make them be honest with you about it. You need to know how your back pain problem has affected them and how it might affect your relationships with them in the future.

The people you are close to need to know from you what you think of them and what your intentions are. You need to talk out problems and frustrations you have with these people. You may not be able to work out all of the differences to your advantage, but you must get your feelings out in the open. The differences need to be understood. Your back pain cannot be a way of communicating those differences or of gaining an advantage, if you are to rid yourself of that pain and the tensions that aggravate it.

Once you are able to evaluate honestly the role that your emotions play and the feelings and expectations of those around you, you are then ready to make decisions about dealing with the problems. Not all of these problems are solvable. You must identify the ones you can solve and put your time and energy into the solutions. Those that are not, you must relax about. If you are making an effort to deal with what can be dealt with and you can openly and honestly share your feelings about what cannot be dealt with, you will have a lot of support. Everyone has weaknesses and problems. People look for others who are willing to share their problems and laugh at them or talk them out.

People don't like to be manipulated by those who are not willing to face the real issues honestly. Most people with chronic pain feel lonely and isolated because others have withdrawn from them. That withdrawal is usually the result of feelings of being manipulated, from feeling that too much is being asked. People with chronic pain who don't confuse the problems of their painful conditions with other psychological needs and who bear their pains without making unnecessary demands on others do not suffer that isolation. What seems to be a simple, easy way to gain some reward by using back pain can have devastating long-range effects. The need to manipulate for a small advantage in dealing with someone can increase gradually and eventually produce an isolation and psychological, if not physical, withdrawal of those who were close.

Pain can become a way of life. A certain amount of advantage in dealing with employers, social agencies, family, or friends may be gained by pain-related behavior. Those who see the whole picture know that, whatever the advantages, they are never worth the price that is paid in the end.

Once the psychological factors are recognized and attempts are made to deal with them honestly and to confront them, the next step is to try to modify pain-induced behavior. People who have accepted the pain way of life build all sorts of habits that depend on pain. Frequently, their spouses or those they work with become involved in these patterns and unwittingly encourage them.

All sorts of little rewards may be taken or given for pain-related behavior. 'Pills with a pleasant psychological side effect or drinks of alcohol are taken when the pain is bad. Anxiety-provoking social contacts are avoided when the pain is bad. Difficult or unpleasant work is not done because the pain is bad. And so on.

Once recognized, these pain games must be changed to wellness games. Deny yourself a drink or a dessert when the pain is there, and reward yourself with one when you have done a hard day's work or have accomplished something you had previously been afraid to try. Talk frankly with those close to you and get them to stop doing you favors when you are having pain and to reward you with some when you are not. Recognize the signals you give that ask for help or for isolation—such things as moans, sighs, grimaces, and holding the sore places. Try to stop doing those things and ask those around you to ignore them.

Some Useful Psychological Gimmicks

The pathway that links psychological difficulty with back pain often involves tension, both in the mental sense and in the sense of tight muscles. Relief from tension may come from use of relaxation techniques. Many of those techniques are directed toward muscle relaxation, and they are described in Chapter 12 as relaxation exercises. Here are some simple self-help gimmicks that are directed more toward the mental aspect of the problem.

It helps to have at hand a list of commandments or aphorisms that you may call upon when situations demand. This may sound a little simplistic and naive, but it can be a very helpful psychological tool. It helps to write them out and carry them with you on a little card until you know them by heart. The following are examples to give you the idea, but you should choose what fits you best and write your own:

I take charge of my own health.
I am polite but open and honest about my feelings.
I talk out my problems with people to whom I am close.

I choose to be healthy.

I can only be in one place at one time.

I do not depend on drugs, alcohol, or nicotine to solve my problems.

I am not perfect, but I am a good person.

Being strong and healthy is better than being weak and sick.

I get better every day.

I do not let my pain be someone else's problem.

Pain doesn't stop me from doing things that are important to me.

A little more sophisticated means of talking to yourself involves the use of what has been called guided imagery. With this technique, you can reeducate your mind to regard the pain in a different way and reduce the fears and other adverse reactions that may accompany pain.

We all recognize that our brains directly and consciously can dictate voluntary activity so that, for example, when the brain says, "Walk," the appropriate leg muscles act and walking results. Sometimes our brains don't act in such concrete, verbal terms; instead, they may react to images. Watching an erotic dance may produce the physical changes of sexual excitement, watching a sad movie may produce tears, and watching someone eat something tasty may result in mouth watering.

When the mind must deal with pain, we know it is not always successful with a direct verbal approach. Telling the pain to go away or telling yourself that the pain isn't there may help a little, but often it won't help much. One of the problems is that pain isn't really out there to take hold of or to speak to directly. Attempts by many people to understand their pains in anatomic or medical terms don't lead to their being able to deal with the pain more effectively.

Many people describe their pains in such terms as "burning pokers," "stabbing knives," or "crushing in a vise." Such terms are the language of imagery, the characterization of an abstract situation by a visual image. Guided imagery is a technique that seeks to encourage the development of such an image and then to attempt to gain mastery over the pain by altering the image.

First, you should practice forming a visual image. Select a picture or furniture object that is available for you to check. Close your eyes, and try to form a mental image of the object. Then, open your eyes and inspect it. Search for every little detail that you may have left out of your image. Repeat this until your image becomes very rich in detail.

Next, get into the rest position or into one of the positions described in Chapter 11. Close your eyes and imagine yourself sitting or lying in some place with which you are very familiar and in which you feel very safe. Form the image of that place in great detail.

Now, allow an image of the pain or the back problem you associate with the pain to appear before you. This may be something very lifelike and representational, such as a rope knot tightening in your back, or it may be something very abstract or fragmented, such as a color or a jagged line.

Relax and allow the image to form. Once it comes, let it evolve and change a bit. Examine it in all its details. Look on every side of it. Observe its color, its texture, its form, its temperature, its smell, its sounds, its movements—everything about it. Relax and examine it without fear and without being attracted to it or repulsed by it. Just examine this image of your pain very carefully.

Next, begin to ask the image of your pain to change in a favorable way. Make it change so that it is less threatening. Allow it to change slowly, to transform into something more manageable. If it is a hot poker, let cool sprinkles of water gradually cool it; if it is a jagged red lightening bolt, let its corners and its point smooth and its color fade into lavender and then blue; if it is a great rope knot in your back, let it slowly untie, and watch the rope fibers break and crumble away.

Once the image has evolved to something manageable and less threatening, let it fade to gray and disappear, let the familiar safe place image return, then open your eyes, stretch, and go on about your day.

By repeating this exercise of guided imagery, you may get in touch with your disorder and your pains in terms that are more understandable to the part of your mind that reacts on a more emotional level. Regarding your problem in this way also gives you the sense of being more in control of your own well-being.

Everyone has psychological and behavioral problems; everyone can do better with them than they do. Simple recognition of those facts and an applied effort start you in the right direction toward a solution. If the problems seem overwhelming and you can make no headway with them, consultation with clergy, a psychologist, or a psychiatrist may help you get started. For most people who can recognize the difficulty and begin to work on it, professional help is not necessary. As with exercise, the important thing is to begin moving in the right direction. Progress may be slow and difficult at times, but continued movement toward solutions will begin to show positive results with long-range benefits.

6
DRUGS AND ALCOHOL

There is a recurrent theme in this book that back pain can usually be managed by self-care measures. Taking prescription medicines is not self-care. It can be done only with reasonable safety under a physician's management. Some people with back pain associated with chronic inflammatory diseases really are benefited by prescription drugs. Others periodically may need prescription drugs for acute flare-ups of pain. Most of the time for most people with back pain, however, drugs are not necessary and may be even harmful. The discussion of prescription drugs in this chapter is offered to give you a more complete understanding of one aspect of back care and thereby make you more competent at self-care. It is certainly not meant to endorse taking prescription drugs as a cure for back pain or to encourage you to rely upon drugs to manage your back pain.

Although alcohol is available without prescription and is not generally considered as a medical drug, its use to relieve back pain is so common and the problems associated with it are so similar to those associated with some prescription drugs used for the same purposes that they will be discussed together.

Opinions about the effects of drugs vary considerably, even among experts. Those given here are from the perspective of a physician who treats people with spinal pain. The drugs named are common examples; they are not meant to comprise a complete list. Specific information about drugs may be obtained from drug information centers or from your doctor or pharmacist.

Recent media attention has been given to the withdrawal of an anti-inflammatory drug called Oraflex and a nonnarcotic analgesic called Zomax from the American market after reports of deaths that seemed to result from taking these drugs. Both of these drugs had been tested extensively before their release. These events testify to the changeable and uncertain nature of drug usage recommendations. No doubt, other drugs, perhaps some that are discussed in this chapter, will be condemned in the future. It would be a great disservice to those who are truly benefited by drug treatments to recommend that no drugs be taken, but these occurrences underscore the need for informed discretion in the use of any medication.

Anti-Inflammatory Medicines

There are a large number of anti-inflammatory drugs. There are two groups—the steroidal or cortisone-like drugs and the nonsteroidal ones that are chemically and biologically unlike cortisone.

Few people with back pain take cortisone over a long period of time. Cortisone shots or short courses of cortisone are reasonably low-risk treatments that, when properly given by a physician, can help control acute symptoms of inflammation. Prolonged taking of cortisone is associated with predictable and severe side effects and must be done only for specific indications under the careful monitoring of a physician.

The nonsteroidal anti-inflammatory drugs are chemically unlike one another and both chemically and biologically unlike cortisone. They share the characteristics of helping to reduce inflammation in joints and connective tissues and of being fairly free of effects on mental status and danger of addiction. Aspirin is the classic example. Acetaminophen (the ingredient in Tylenol and Datril) is not included in this group. Phenyl-butazone (Butazolidin, Azolid), oxyphenbutazone (Tandearil), sulindac (Clinoril), indomethacin (Indocin), meclofenamate (Meclomen), mefenamic acid (Ponstel), ibuprofen (Motrin, Rufen), fenoprofen (Nal-fon), naproxen (Naprosyn), tolmetin (Tolectin), and piroxican (Feldene) are commonly prescribed members of this group. Colchicine, a drug commonly used to relieve inflammation caused by gout, also is pre-scribed sometimes to control inflammatory responses to spinal disorders other than gout. Except for aspirin and colchicine, these drugs are all fairly expensive. They are all associated with potentially serious side effects, though for those who are helped by them the risk is acceptably low to warrant long-term use. Many people are not helped by these drugs or have side effects, such as stomach upset, which make them intolerant of these drugs. Of course, those people should not take them.

Aspirin, because of its effectiveness, relative inexpensiveness and availability, and long-term widespread usage, is still the most popular of these drugs. It may not always be the most effective or best tolerated for a given individual, however. To make it more tolerable, a large number of coated and chemically altered forms of salicylates are available, such as Ascriptin, Arthropan, Bufferin, Ecotrin, Trilisate, Dolobid, Zorprin, and various brands of sodium salicylate, magnesium salicylate, and sodium thiosalicylate. These coated and altered forms of aspirin cause stomach upset and gastrointestinal bleeding less often than aspirin but they are more expensive. Aspirin in any form aggravates asthma or allergic nasal stuffiness in about 10 percent of people who suffer from those problems.

Muscle Relaxants

The group of drugs called muscle relaxants is chemically an oddly diverse group of drugs that are prescribed frequently in combined forms with common anti-inflammatories and pain relievers. Pharmacologically, it is doubtful that these drugs really have a primary effect of relaxing muscles, and clinically there seems to be little difference between the responses of people to these drugs and the responses to nonnarcotic analgesics.

Whether these drugs have any primary effect of muscle relaxation or the muscle relaxation achieved just occurs because of pain relief or sedative effects of these medications, the term *muscle relaxant* is generally understood by those who deal with these problems to mean one of a group of drugs of generally low addiction and side effect potential that may provide some relief from musculoskeletal pain. The effects and the precautions in use are essentially the same as for the anti-inflammatories and nonnarcotic pain relievers. To treat this as a distinct class of drugs makes little sense from a clinical point of view, but common use and the influence of promotional advertising perpetuates the practice.

Commonly used examples, including the combination forms, are chlorphenesin (Maolate), orphenadrine (Norflex, Norgesic), chloroxazone (Paraflex, Parafon), methocarbamol (Robaxin, Robaxisal), metaxalone (Skelaxin), and carisoprodol (Soma, Soma Compound).

Cyclobenzaprine (Flexeril) is chemically and therapeutically so similar to the tricyclic group of drugs considered under antidepressants that it is best considered in that discussion.

Another drug commonly promoted and used as a muscle relaxant is diazepam (Valium), a drug with such potent antianxiety effects and side effects that, along with similar drugs, it is best considered with the discussion of tranquilizers. The same may be said for meprobamate (Equanil, Miltown, Equagesic), which also is used sometimes for muscle relaxation.

Tranquilizers

Drugs considered as tranquilizers all have the effect of altering mental status and have some addiction potential. Most tranquilizers have a "downer" effect, which helps to relieve anxiety and nervousness. Many are not unlike alcohol in that they have a rapid initial calming effect and a long-range danger of depression and habituation.

Few people become addicted to these drugs in the sense that addiction can develop to narcotic pain relievers. Many people, however, become habituated to them. These drugs provide what seems to be some relief for a short time, but they undermine the will and determination to get to the real problems with real solutions and, except for very short-term use for acute anxiety, they do little real good for people with back pain.

Phenobarbital is the classic example of this type of drug. Because it and other barbiturates have been used and misused for a long time, the hazards are commonly known and, thus, it is not prescribed as often as it once was. Other, newer drugs with somewhat similar effects and hazards are in very common use. The hazards, of course, depend on dosage, frequency of ingestion, and number of days of use.

Meprobamate (Equanil, Miltown), hydroxyzine (Atarax, Vistaril), and the benzodiazepines (Librium, Serax, Tranxene, Ativan, Centrax, Valium) are commonly used drugs of this group. Because of its widespread use to control many anxiety, pain, and tension-related symptoms, diazepam (Valium) is probably the drug of this type that is most commonly abused to the detriment of back pain sufferers. The result of prolonged use is drug dependency, diminished energy and motivation, depression, and reduced pain tolerance. Diazepam deserves the criticism it has received in those regards but probably no more so than less famous drugs of the same group. All of the tranquilizing drugs have the potential to produce harmful side effects when taken for chronic pain. There are specific indications for the use of these drugs, and they should be taken only under the management of a physician who is aware of what other medicines are being taken and what other problems are present (most particularly, the problem of controlling chronic back pain).

There are many other drugs used to relieve anxiety. Some of these are sometimes called major tranquilizers and are more often used when there is a major primary problem with anxiety or thought disorder. They are most commonly prescribed by a psychiatrist or a physician experienced in the management of their effects. The largest group of these drugs is called phenothiazines, common examples being Thorazine, Haldol, Stelazine, and Mellaril. These drugs may be used in small doses to control more ordinary anxiety problems, are sometimes combined with antidepressants, and may be used to control such diverse problems as nausea and sleeplessness. Even in small doses and less active forms, these drugs have the potential to produce very serious side effects and should never be taken except according to a physician's prescription.

Antidepressants

Several drugs are used primarily to control depression. Some of these have been found to be effective in the control of chronic pain. Whether the pain seems less bad as the depression is relieved, the relief of depression allows for a more healthful life style resulting in fewer pain-producing stimuli, or some intermediate phase of the chain of transmission from stimulus to conscious pain perception is altered by these drugs is not completely understood. All of these modes of action may work together. Regardless, the observation made is that many people with chronic pain seem to improve after taking one of these medications for a period of time. The positive effects are not rapid as they are with analgesic and tranquilizing medications.

Many of the antidepressant drugs commonly used to control pain are sometimes referred to as tricyclics because of the shape of the chemical representation of the basic molecule. Common examples are amitriptyline (Elavil, Amitid, Endep), doxepin (Adapin, Sinequan), amoxapine (Ascendin), nortriptyline (Aventyl, Pamelor), protriptyline (Vivactil), maprotiline (Ludiomil), desipramine (Norpramin, Pertofrane), and imipramine (Tofranil). Chemically distinct but clinically similar is trazodone (Desyrel). These drugs may be prepared in combination with tranquilizers (Deprol, Limbitrol, Etrafon, Triavil).

Many people experience unpleasant physical side effects from these drugs, such as dry mouth, visual blurring, and increased appetite, and unpleasant mental side effects, such as bad dreams, sedation, or nervousness. There is much individual variation in response to these drugs, so the safest and most effective use may require careful monitoring, including blood testing, under the supervision of a physician who is expert in their use. This is more apt to be necessary for patients who are going to try to take the drug in spite of side effects, or who have a major primary problem with depression.

Pain Relievers

Medicines called pain relievers vary enormously in their modes of action, their effects, and their dangers. Nonsteroidal anti-inflammatory drugs may be used effectively for pain relief since much musculoskeletal pain is the result of inflammation. Acetaminophen is one of the safest pain-relieving medications and is available without prescription and at reasonable cost.

Propoxyphene (Darvon) is an intermediate-strength pain reliever with mild addiction potential and slightly greater risk of side effects. Though most people have no problem with it, a few become habituated to propoxyphene and develop a strong desire for increasing doses of the drug. It is frequently combined with aspirin (Darvon Compound) or acetaminophen (Darvocet, Wygesic) to increase its effectiveness. Taking it with alcohol or other potent drugs may increase substantially the dangers of its use.

Ethoheptazine (Zactane) is another commonly used nonnarcotic pain reliever with the same general properties as propoxyphene. It also is combined commonly with aspirin (Zactirin).

The nonsteroidal anti-inflammatory drugs have either a direct or an indirect (or both) effect on pain relief. An anti-inflammatory preparation (Motrin, Nalfon, various salicylates) or a chemical derivation of one (Anaprox, Ponstel) may be prescribed as a pain reliever.

Many over-the-counter and some prescription drugs used as pain relievers are really combinations of tranquilizers, anti-inflammatories, stimulants (caffeine), and pain relievers. Commonly prescribed examples include Equagesic (meprobamate, ethoheptazine, and aspirin). Fiorinal (butalbital, aspirin, phenacetin, and caffeine), Synalgos (promethazine, aspirin, phenacetin, and caffeine), and Zactirin Compound (ethoheptazine, aspirin, phenacetin, and caffeine).

Pain relievers that contain codeine have more addiction potential than the drugs discussed above. Like all narcotic drugs, they become less effective the more they are used. They have the unpleasant side effect of constipation. Codeine, too, is frequently combined with other drugs to increase its potency and decrease the dosage needed for the desired effect. Aspirin (Empirin with Codeine, Ascodeine), acetaminophen (Empracet with Codeine, Phenaphen with Codeine, Tylenol with Codeine), and multiple ingredient combinations (Fiorinal with Codeine) frequently are designated with the following numbers: 2 meaning 15 milligrams of codeine, 3 for 30 milligrams of codeine, and 4 signifying 60 milligrams (or one grain) of codeine.

Synthetically made drugs very similar, chemically and biologically, to codeine have been developed in an attempt to provide increased effects with decreased side effects. In the commonly used doses and combination forms, these drugs seem to have more addiction potential than the commonly used doses and forms of codeine. At least the number of patients with back pain who have developed a harmful dependency on narcotic drugs seems to be greater with these codeine derivatives than it does with codeine itself. Oxycodone (Percodan, Percocet, Tylox) is the most commonly abused of these drugs. Hydrocodone (Vicodin) and dihydrocodone (Synalgos DC) are other examples of this type of drug.

Pentazocine (Talwin) is an intermediate-strength narcotic drug similar in strength and addiction potential to but chemically unlike the codeine drugs. It should not be used except in short-term, acute pain situations.

Morphine, oxymorphone (Numorphan), hydromorphone (Dilaudid), and meperidine (Demerol, Mepergan) are strong narcotic medications that should be used for back pain only in very unusual circumstances and then almost always in a hospital or a very controlled situation.

Alcohol

Having considered the different types and classes of back pain medicine, I would like to return to further discussion of alcohol. Alcohol is very commonly misused for relief of back pain and other chronic pain conditions.

The reason why people become habituated to the use of alcohol for control of pain is very similar to the reason why many become habituated to the use of some of the drugs just described. The drugs most often involved in this phenomenon are alcohol, tranquilizers, and codeine derivatives. Use of these drugs together or in combination is particularly dangerous.

People who use alcohol habitually to relieve pain or who rely heavily on tranquilizers, codeine derivatives, or some combination of these drugs have more trouble ridding themselves of back pain than any other single group of patients, regardless of the anatomic origin of the pain.

If you rely heavily on alcohol with or without other drugs to control back pain, it is absolutely necessary that you free yourself from that burden if you are ever to be free of the back pain. For some people, the primary problem is alcohol or drug dependency. Some people have a constitution that makes them so susceptible to the addictive potential of alcohol or certain drugs that they must consider themselves allergic to them and must avoid absolutely any contact with them. Their health and indeed their lives depend on avoiding the alcohol or drug.

Some people already caught in the trap of such alcohol or drug dependency find that escape from back pain becomes a reason to go on taking the drug. Others may never have been aware of their susceptibility to alcohol or drugs and only experience the difficulty after they have developed a spinal problem and begin to use alcohol or drugs for back pain. Once you are caught in this web of habituation, your mind's craving for the drug becomes so strong that the pain appears as a signal and justification for more drugs.

There is no escaping the cycle of back pain and dependency on alcohol and addictive drugs without withdrawal from the drugs and alcohol. The idea that the drugs or alcohol will be given up as soon as something is done to fix the back never works. If alcohol or drug addiction is already a problem, it needs to be discussed frankly with doctor, spouse, and those who care. Professional help may be needed. If there is only a suggestion that alcohol or drug dependency could be part of the problem, the alcohol or drug dependency needs to be cut off immediately.

Most people can tolerate an occasional drink of alcohol without serious consequence. For those who can tolerate it, alcohol can serve as a tension reliever. When alcohol interferes with meaningful function and responsibilities or when it interferes with meaningful communication with loved ones, it should be avoided altogether.

For those who have back pain, particular care must be taken to avoid using alcohol as a pain reliever. The records of those who have tried provide overwhelming evidence of the danger and lack of success of this method of back pain control.

If you have enough experience with alcohol to know that it brings you pleasure safely and without risk of making things worse for yourself, you may be able to use it to your advantage. Deprive yourself of alcohol when you are down with back pain—you must do that anyway to avoid the risk of using it for back pain. Reward yourself with a drink if you are feeling well or if you have made some substantial progress in returning to a normal life.

The above endorsement of the use of alcohol is a very qualified one. No one who does not have a history of successful use of alcohol without ill effects should ever begin to use it when having any trouble with his or her health, including back pain. Alcohol should not be used by anyone taking any pain-relieving or tranquilizing medicine. Alcohol should never be taken in excess. Alcohol should never be used to relieve back pain or symptoms associated with spinal disorders. If alcohol is used at all, it should be used infrequently, in small doses, and at times when symptoms are diminished and function improved.

Natural Pain Relievers

There is an increasing amount of scientific information about hormones that the body produces to provide pain relief or resistance to pain. There is still much to be understood about these natural pain-control hormones, called endorphins.

Your body will produce more of these pain-resisting hormones if you exercise vigorously on a regular basis as discussed in Chapter 11.

The natural production of these hormones may be suppressed by taking pain medicines. That may explain why medicines don't help much after a while and why pain gets worse temporarily if regular medicines are stopped. This mechanism would explain the common observation that regular reliance on medicine to control chronic back pain often only makes things worse and why, given enough time, fitness exercise makes things better.

7
NUTRITION AND WEIGHT CONTROL

Your health and feeling of well-being are related to proper nutrition. A fast-paced lifestyle and dependency on processed foods result in nutritional deficiencies for many people. However, in developed nations, the most common diet problem related to back pain is the consumption of too many calories.

Nutrition

In spite of agricultural riches and high standards of living, many Americans and citizens of other highly-developed nations are nutritionally deprived. Dependency on fast, processed foods may result in vitamin and mineral deficiencies. The idea of needing large amounts of protein has resulted in diets too rich in the saturated fats which accompany protein-rich foods such as red meats. Each year the average American consumes 15 pounds of salt (about 30 times what is needed) and 128 pounds of sugar. Salt and sugar are necessary to preserve processed foods and to make them palatable. Saturated fats contribute to cardiovascular disease and salt to high blood pressure. Sugar provides calories without contributing to other nutritional needs.

People who do not take particular care to ensure that they receive a well-balanced diet are likely to feel hungry and dissatisfied much of the time because the simple sugars they ingest are absorbed rapidly, resulting in rapid swings of blood sugar and feelings of emptiness in the abdomen. They try to dispel those feelings by eating more sugary and salted foods. They eat too much meat and other fatty foods and not enough of the complex carbohydrates obtained from such foods as potatoes and whole grains. They do not eat enough unprocessed fruits and vegetables to maintain an adequate intake of vitamins and minerals. They do not obtain enough fiber from their diets.

The best approach to this problem is to learn about proper nutrition and follow good nutritional practices. For those who are uncertain about the adequacy of their diets and cannot make sure they have balanced diets, it is worthwhile to take a daily multiple vitamin-mineral supplement. People who have been ill, are on weight-reduction diets, or are otherwise unusually stressed, are advised to do so especially.

Calcium-deficient diets are very common. Many people have a progressive weakening of their bones as they age, to the point where their bones may fracture from trivial injury. This problem is called *osteoporosis*. Complications of osteoporosis are common causes of back pain among older people. One of the factors which contributes to osteoporosis is calcium deficiency. It is especially common in women after the menopause. Unless they drink several glasses of milk (skimmed milk is best) each day or eat large amounts of other calcium-rich foods, women should take calcium supplements during and after menopause. Most diets contain only about 500 mg of calcium per day. The minimum daily requirement is often stated to be 800 mg, but may be as high as 1500 mg for postmenopausal women.

Other than a supplement to provide minimum daily requirements of vitamins and minerals, special diet-supplements are not necessary to prevent or treat back pain. It is particularly useless and unfortunate for people to spend money and place their hopes on special diet and vitamin cures for back pain and related complaints involving musculoskeletal discomfort. These "cures" represent well-meaning but misguided attempts to buy an easy way out of problems that must be attacked by learning proper care, exercise, and stress control. Unfortunately, the latter requires a lot of dedication and effort whereas the former only requires some money, swallowing a few pills, or eating some unusual diet combinations. The problem is that the dedicated effort approach really helps, and the fad diets and pills only lead to frustration.

What Should You Weigh?

Being overweight causes increased difficulty with back pain because it adversely affects spinal posture, results in increased mechanical stress to vulnerable parts of the spinal anatomy, interferes with efforts at normal movement and exercise, and depletes energy and the feeling of well-being. An individual's ideal weight may depend on many factors. No one, however, has back pain because he or she carries too little excess fat.

Most well-conditioned athletes weigh much less than their nonathletic counterparts, even in spite of the extra muscle weight they carry. Exceptions that occur in well-publicized sports like football are because the sports attract heavily built individuals, the athletes' muscle development is extreme, or, in some cases, extra weight is carried intentionally. Runners, swimmers, tennis players, basketball players, and most other athletes, in contrast, weigh a good bit less than nonathletes of the same height.

The lean, conditioned body weight of most men of 66 to 72 inches in height is between 135 and 175 pounds. Some men may wish to carry more weight because they think it looks good or helps them in some way, but if the goal is to keep body weight and excess fat down to relieve or prevent back pain, few men should carry more than 175 pounds.

The ideal weight of most 20-year-old women between 60- and 70-inches tall is from 105 to 135 pounds. Ideal weights are adjusted up with advancing age so that 60-year-olds should be about 15 pounds heavier than 20-year-olds. The thin look of most models and actresses more nearly approximates the ideal healthy body build for women than does the macho, heavily built image of football players for men. Thinness should not be achieved, however, at the expense of adequate nutrition and muscle development. Muscle is not unhealthy and is necessary to protect you from injuries which cause back pain. Weight reduction at the expense of muscle mass is unhealthful. Recent medical evidence supports the contention that a little excess body fat is more healthful than extreme leanness, but that evidence should not be cited to justify obesity.

What is or is not attractive about thinness and fat is certainly open to question. Many people think they and their loved ones look healthier, more robust, more successful, and happier if they carry some excess fat. Maintaining that look, however, may be a luxury that is not worth the cost for people with back pain.

If you count up all of the miles you walk, the stairs you climb, and the distance your body weight is raised and lowered when you get into and out of beds, chairs, automobiles, and so on, and multiply that by the weight of your body, you will see that you do an astounding number of foot-pounds of work. Reduction of your body weight by only a few pounds, therefore, can reduce substantially the stresses that are placed on your body even by ordinary activity. Besides any local stresses to the back, the general fatigue caused by carrying extra fat around aggravates the pain and saps the energy needed to enjoy healthful activities.

Body weight is not, however, the only important determinant of the effect obesity may have on back pain. The distribution of excess weight may be even more important than the number of pounds of it. Some overweight people have heavy legs and a flat abdomen; others are the opposite. It is when the excess weight is carried in the abdomen that it is most likely to cause trouble with back pain.

Abdomens become big in overweight people because of fat deposited in the subcutaneous tissues between the skin and the muscles of the abdomen and also because of fat deposited in the omentum, lying on the intestines within the abdominal cavity. Both areas of abdominal fat deposits cause problems that lead to back pain.

The fat inside the abdomen stretches the abdominal muscles, robbing them of their tone. The spine and the short, heavy muscles of the back prevent the overfilled abdomen from stretching out in back, so it stretches out frontward, over the belt. The fat in the subcutaneous tissues adds extra weight and bulk to the very front of the abdomen.

Excessive abdominal fat thus results in a forward shift of the body's center of gravity, the central axis of the body's weight around which the spine and muscles must support the body to keep it upright. The stretched-out abdominal muscles are less able to pull the center of gravity back toward the spine to exert pressure through the abdomen to support the spine.

The only way the lumbar spine can accommodate this additional stress is to sway further—to go into more lordosis, so as to tip the upper body backward. Otherwise, the body would topple forward. As the upper body is tipped backward, the head and shoulders are allowed to slump forward to balance the upper body and bring the eye level straight ahead.

The results of the excessive lordosis caused by abdominal obesity are more stress and more back pain because the facets override and the nerves are pinched as they emerge from the spine. One answer to these problems is abdominal muscle strengthening exercise to recover lost tone and build extra strength to support the spine. The other answer is weight reduction.

Excess weight does not cause normal discs to rupture. It does cause and aggravate the back pain that usually accompanies disc trouble. It contributes to mechanical back pains, which may be very similar to the pains that occur from ruptured discs. Weight reduction by itself is not apt to cure back pain completely, but it helps, and without it complete relief is less attainable.

Weight Reduction Diets

How do you lose weight? For people who recognize that they have been eating too much, the answer is obvious. However, many overweight people honestly believe that they do not overeat and some of them have good reason to believe that. They may eat far less than thin spouses or friends. They may consume fewer calories than what is said to be right for them.

For some people, it just isn't fair. There is no answer to that, but fair or not, those people can still lose weight.

If you reduce your calorie intake enough, you can lose weight. You may have to reduce your calorie intake far more than other people to achieve the same reduction. You may have to keep it reduced for longer than some others to make the same progress. Sometimes weight loss is unexplainably uneven, with no loss at all for days or weeks, then loss for a while, and then another plateau of no loss.

Diet pills may be unsafe, ineffective, or both. They have the bad effect of displacing the responsibility for weight control, and with that they rob you of the sense of personal achievement you feel from your success. They may also increase feelings of tension and anxiety. The control must come from your determination, not from a pill.

The essential features of any diet that works are that total calorie consumption must be reduced and the diet must be acceptably safe and tolerable for permanent maintenance.

Extreme, fad diets that severely limit food choices or that are overloaded with certain food types while depriving you of others may work temporarily, either because they are bad nutritionally or because they are so unpalatable that the real effect is to reduce calorie intake drastically.

Some popular diets that provide good nutrition and then have a built-in mechanism to guide the dieter to a permanent maintenance diet that is palatable and nutritious are acceptable. The enthusiasm generated by their proponents and the opportunity to follow them with someone else are big plus factors that may help you get started.

Diets that promise to take several pounds off very rapidly may have an appeal, but that is the wrong appeal. If you are overweight, you have probably been so for a long time, and you have probably gradually become more so. What you want is to reverse that direction permanently, to begin losing instead of gaining, and to keep losing until you reach a lean body build. Then you want to stay there, never again to go back in the direction of gaining.

You want a diet that promises you only that—adequate nutrition and a permanent change from the direction of gaining to that of losing, then maintenance without ever changing back to the direction of gaining. You don't care how fast you get there as long as you keep going in the right direction.

Accept the important principles of weight reduction. Even if you are one of those people for whom it isn't fair because you don't lose weight in spite of a reasonably low calorie intake, if your calorie intake is low enough for long enough, you will lose weight. Your diet change must provide adequate nutrition, it must be palatable, and it must be permanent. If you adhere to those principles, you will succeed. Beyond that commitment, there are a number of safe tricks that make it easier to control your weight.

Understanding Hunger

If you analyze what makes you want to eat, you may be able to establish a healthier diet pattern. Most people assume that they eat because they are hungry and that the hunger is their body's way of telling them they need more nutrition. In fact, it is rare that most people in developed nations are in any real nutritional need for more calories. As successful dieters and athletes on high energy expenditure, low-calorie regimens find, the real calorie needs of our bodies are a great deal less than what most people consume. That is why even quite a substantial reduction of calorie intake often will not lead to weight loss. If the number of calories is reduced enough for long enough, however, weight will always come off.

If we don't eat because we need nutrition, then why do we get hungry? Of course, partaking of food that smells and tastes good is one of life's great pleasures, but many people who enjoy that pleasure don't eat too much. Most people who do overeat recognize that they eat too fast or too much to be really savoring the tastes and smells.

From the first moments of life, we associate eating with comfort and attention. It is not surprising, then, that when we feel depressed, lonely, bored, or frustrated, one of the first things we feel is hunger and one of the first places we turn is to the refrigerator. Eating seldom helps for more than a few minutes, though, and for those who are overweight, the guilt feelings that follow often just make the depression and frustration greater.

Many people eat when they are angry. Anger with a spouse, kids, boss, or loved one that is not expressed directly sometimes results in frustrations that lead to diet abuse. Many people do things to damage themselves when they are angered by someone else, and one of the most popular ways to accomplish that is overeating.

Many people eat in response to these emotions from habit. Few people consciously think, "I am hungry; therefore, I will eat," or, "I am bored; therefore, I will eat." Most people who eat for those reasons do it because of unconscious, repeated patterns of behavior.

You may be able to recognize the things that make you hungry if, for a few days, you keep a list of exactly what you eat and when and what you are doing and feeling at the time you eat. Patterns may emerge that help you to see why you overeat better than you ever could see by trying to figure it out one snack at a time.

When you make such a list, you may discover that you have been eating a great deal more than you had realized. Another thing that sometimes happens is that making the list becomes part of the cure. If you know you have to confess to it by writing it down, you may decide it isn't worth it and pass it up.

Exercise and Weight Control

To combine exercise with a low-calorie diet is a popular and valid approach to losing excess weight. However, many misconceptions exist about the effects of exercise on attempts at weight reduction. Many people say that they should lose weight because they get a lot of exercise while doing their jobs, or they say that they must "eat well" because they get so much exercise or do so much work. People who believe those things often take in too many calories, and the misconceptions they have about exercise make their weight problems worse.

In fact, it is almost impossible to lose weight by exercise alone. Only very extreme amounts of exercise, such as that obtained by long-distance runners who stay in condition for marathon running, ever seem to have a substantial direct effect on weight. Even then, the contribution of exercise is only partial, because the thinness those people maintain is partially the result of the fact that they usually consume fewer calories than overweight people who are less physically active. Contrary to what many think, people who get extreme amounts of exercise usually have smaller appetites than other people and smaller appetites than they themselves have when they do not get regular, vigorous exercise.

The actual calories burned even by vigorous exercise or by working hard all day are surprisingly few. If such activity is used as an excuse for diet abuse, the effect of exercise on an attempt to lose weight may be negative. If you resist the temptation, however, exercise can benefit your weight reduction efforts in other ways.

Regular exercise requires some reordering of the day's activities. Those changes in routine can include avoidance of some of the temptations to eat. Eating just before exercise is undesirable because it may cause abdominal cramps, discomfort, or nausea while exercising. Right after exercise, most people do not feel like eating or can have their needs met by a low-calorie drink. It may be best to schedule your exercise purposely at times when you would be most tempted to go off your diet.

Exercise usually improves regular bowel function. That relieves the tendency to overeat or snack in search of relief from vague feelings of discomfort in the abdomen.

For people who eat because they are depressed, bored, frustrated, or angry, while some of those problems may require more direct attack on the source of the trouble, it is best to find some displacement activity other than eating to dispel those feelings. Exercise works exceptionally well for that purpose.

People who exercise regularly feel healthy and strong. They do not want to abuse their bodies by overeating.

Besides coordinating your diet with exercise, you can employ a number of other helpful and harmless steps to make your weight reduction effort more successful or at least less painful:

Eat only at regular meals.

Avoid coffee and alcohol before meals.

Eat only at one or two places.

Don't read or watch TV during meals.

Use a small plate.

Take small bites. Use a small spoon.

Concentrate on the tastes and smells as you eat.

Talk at mealtime only when your mouth is empty.

Completely empty your mouth before taking another bite.

Put eating utensils down between bites.

Eat the best things first.

Wait 20 minutes before taking a second serving.

Don't eat scraps left at the end of meals.

Change your routine to avoid situations where you eat.

If you must snack, plan and prepare it in advance.

Don't snack while you are doing something else.

Don't snack while watching TV—try knitting or carving.

Don't leave goodies sitting out (such as in cookie jars).

Refrigerate goodies in opaque containers at the back of the frig.

Drink plenty of water, especially before meals.

Eat high fiber foods.

Drink skimmed milk.

Use oil and vinegar rather than cheese or cream dressings.

Bake, boil, and broil rather than fry.

Use whipped margarine.

Avoid simple sugars such as candy, cookies, and soft drinks.

Do your kids and yourself a favor by not keeping sugar goodies.

Eat at the salad bars if you must go to fast food restaurants.

Assign yourself something else to do when hungry—perhaps exercise.

If you blow it once, take the loss and recoup, don't binge.

Keeping It Off

Most people who are overweight have been on many diets and already know these and other hints very well. What is wrong is that whenever you go on a diet, there is the implication that someday you will go off it, and when you do, you are likely to gain back whatever you lost and then some.

What is needed is a permanent change in diet, a change in what you eat and why you eat. You must eat for adequate nutrition and for the enjoyment of food in limited amounts. You cannot eat to resolve anger, frustration, or vague feelings of discontent, or for more than basic nutritional needs. No matter how low the calorie intake has to go to keep you lean, you must keep it there—even if that doesn't seem fair compared to other people.

You will find that a successful diet and a slim physique are their own rewards. But give yourself a little extra—put aside the money you would have spent on what you didn't eat, make a bet with your spouse, or have a contest with someone else who needs to lose, so that as you reach milestones in attaining your goal, you can present yourself with extra awards.

8
<u>SEX</u>

Backache is second only to headache as a reason given by a marriage partner for not wanting to have sexual intercourse. Many of the reasons why back pain and avoidance of sexual activity might be associated have been touched upon already in this text, but, since this is such an important part of life for so many people and since back pain sufferers often state that it is a problem, it will be worth some repetition.

Body Mechanics of Sex

Certain positions and movements commonly used in the sex act can be physically stressful to the back. Classical sexual intercourse position and movement may lead to forceful hyperextenion of the lumbar spine, which could be painful in some back conditions. Any extreme or unusual posture might become exaggerated to the point of causing back pain during the passion of sexual activity. The muscle tension associated with sexual excitement may add increased stress to already stressful postures.

There are, however, positions for sexual intercourse that result in little stress to the low back. In fact, the positions of rest and postural exercise that you learned elsewhere in this text can be duplicated during sexual intercourse.

The partner with the back problem can lie on the back, a pillow can be placed under the hips and lower back, and knees can be bent—a satisfactory position for sexual intercourse and an ideal position for a sore back. The woman can lie on her side with knees and hips flexed and the man in the same position behind her—again, a satisfactory position for sex and an ideal one for back support and relaxation.

The same position and movement recommendations that are given in the chapters on posture, body mechanics, and exercise apply to sex as they would to any other activity.

Risk of back pain associated with sexual activity is related only to the positions and movements of the back. There is nothing about erection and ejaculation that is stressful to the male back, and if those things are truly painful, a checkup of the prostate and genitourinary organs is in order. Likewise, for women, there is nothing about penetration of the female pelvis that should cause trouble with the back, and if penetration does cause pain consistently in the vagina, pelvis, or back, a consultation for a pelvic examination is needed.

Other Causes of Pain from Sex

Most people find that sexual excitement relieves them from other pains and tensions. Many people find that sleep comes easily after sexual activity. If sex can release people from tension and pain and allow them to relax, and if sex can be accomplished safely by those with back pain, why then is pain from sex or avoidance of sex such a common complaint among back pain sufferers? To answer that question, we must leave the consideration of the back as an anatomic structure and return to look at the full picture of people with back pain.

The anatomic changes that lead some people to have back pain usually progress more rapidly during their thirties, forties, and fifties. Those are times of many stresses and frustrations, including difficult sexual adjustment.

The sexual desire of earlier years is linked in part to desire for reproduction. Once enough children have been born, fear of additional unwanted pregnancies may lead to a desire to avoid sex or fear of sex. For those who have not been able to have children, who have had difficult pregnancies or gynecologic problems, or who have had unsuccessful marriages, the anxieties of those situations may be associated with sex and may lead to avoidance or fear of sex. The romance of early relationships pales with familiarity and repetition and is diluted in importance by worries about kids, jobs, and finances. With the loss of romance, the feeling of sexual attractiveness diminishes and, with it, the desire for sex. People who don't feel sexually attractive don't want sex, just like people who don't feel that they are good at a job or sport don't want to engage in them.

In middle age, people often gain weight, lose muscle power and tone, get wrinkles in their skin, and otherwise show signs of aging. Television, magazines, and movies portray a certain image of what is supposed to be sexually attractive. As the changes in middle age occur, people are less and less able to copy the images that the media set for sexual attractiveness. As we become less like what is supposed to be sexy, we become more afraid and reluctant about our own sexuality.

Many are burdened with the demands of financial obligation, caught in jobs where they don't have the power they would like to have, and, seeing their physical strength and resilience diminish, have some problems with consistent sexual function.

Sex may be the dominant force in the lives of young, energetic people who want to reproduce and are less burdened with the stresses of middle age. As sex becomes a less dominant force, the enjoyment and successful performance of the sex act often diminishes or becomes inconsistent.

Most men experience occasional loss of sexual power—they become unable to obtain or hold an erection during attempts at sexual intercourse. These are normal occurrences. They are often frightening to men and make them feel inadequate or powerless. They may make women feel undesired. These normal occurrences should not have the psychological effects that they do. The most common reason for repeated occurrence of sexual impotence is fear of its occurrence. The anxiety associated with the fear that impotence will occur again makes it much more likely to happen again.

Sexual participation has always been a way in which people show love and appreciation for each other. Unfortunately, the reverse is true also—denial of sexual participation has always been a way for people to express anger and disappointment to each other. If one partner finds it difficult to say, "I'm angry with you," what is said instead (by action if not by words) is, "I won't have sex with you," or if he or she needs to cover the true feelings even more, "I won't have sex with you because my back hurts."

So, back pain as a reason for not having sex can help avoid fears of pregnancy, avoid the fears of unsatisfactory sexual performance, avoid unpleasant memories that may have become associated with sex, avoid verbally expressing disappointment and anger, and work in many like ways to fulfill some psychological need of the moment. Pains and illnesses such as back pain may be used for this purpose, especially at a time of life when sexual desire may have decreased some anyway because of feelings of lost romance and unattractiveness, worries over other important facets of life, or feelings of powerlessness and depression.

So, back pain can be used to avoid an activity that may not seem very desirable at the time anyway, may carry some threat to the ego, and may be symbolic of giving love and affection when the dominant feeling is anger and frustration.

Back pain works for this—for the moment. But what is the price, at the moment and in the longer range? The person with back pain suffers the loss of the release and fulfillment associated with sex. Further estrangement from the partner occurs, not only because the sexual pleasure has been denied but also because it has been denied in a way that is not totally honest. That estrangement results in more frustration, more tension, more stress, more back pain. There follows a temptation to further exaggerate the incapacity caused by the back pain in order to save face.

What Can Be Done?

The most important part of the solution is to recognize the problem. An honest consideration of all of the feelings you may have about sex and your sex partner and of all of the fears you associate with performance and consequences of sex is the first step.

You need to know not only how you think and feel about these things but also how your sex partner regards them. You both need to know how those feelings affect you and how they affect your partner. Many people find it difficult to talk to each other about sex problems. Talking about them is an absolute necessary part of the remedy. Such talk is not only necessary to the full recognition of the problem, but it is also a big part of the solution. If you find it impossible to begin by talking to your partner, begin by talking to someone else. Confide in a friend. You may be surprised to find that there is nothing very unusual about these problems. Most people experience them in one way or another and are glad to have someone to discuss them with honestly. If you are unsuccessful in that, professional counseling from clergy, marriage counselors, psychologists, or psychiatrists can help. The essential fact, though, is that the talk can't stop with a professional or a friend; it must come back to a full honest disclosure of feelings between you and your partner.

Sexual desires do wax and wane. There are times when people don't feel sexy. Partners need to recognize that about each other, talk about it, be considerate with each other, and make reasonable compromises without using false reasons for feelings.

Some women have good reasons to fear pregnancy or pelvic disorders. Their partners need to know about these fears and be supportive in seeking medical solutions or reassurances. Men do have times when they cannot obtain or hold an erection or when they ejaculate prematurely. They need to know about how that makes them feel and listen to their partner talk about how it makes her feel, and then each needs to reassure the other that these things sometimes occur normally and that a relaxed attitude about them is the best measure.

Feelings of anger and disappointment need to be talked out, not acted out through withdrawal from participation in sex or other activities of life. This talking out of anger is so difficult for many people that they have become accustomed to using other methods to vent their anger. They are not consciously aware that what they are doing is motivated by frustration and anger.

Open talk about anger and disappointment between partners can be risky. Fear of being able to control the anger or fear of the partner's reaction are major reasons why the true feelings are often suppressed. These fears are almost always greater than what actually happens— another example of how fear of something going wrong guarantees that something will go wrong and stands in the way of progress. The true feelings really haven't been suppressed but only disguised in actions that are much more damaging than words—to both partners.

9
RECREATION

People need to have fun. To deny yourself the activities in life that bring pleasure is to deprive yourself of the joy of life. Pleasure, to be sure, is gained from work, sex, and interpersonal relationships, but people need some additional, occasional pleasures outside these more regular occurrences.

What you should choose for recreation depends upon your taste and experience. Some activities, of course, are more stressful to your back than others. A few sports carry such high risks of back injury that they are not advisable for people with back trouble. Sports that risk sudden violent stress to the low back are those that should be avoided. Wrestling, trampolining, tumbling, and vigorous contact sports such as football and hockey are examples. The problem with these activities is that there is very little capacity to control the intensity or avoid the possibility of sudden injury. Many other sports have some potential for back injury, but the risks are under much greater control. If you can avoid the possibility of sudden violent stress, the other factors to consider are the intensity and the duration of effort. These two factors can be controlled in most sports at least to some degree. The greatest control is possible in the activities that will be discussed in the section on general fitness exercises in Chapter 11. No other sports can be done with the same benefit and degree of safety as those can, but with some intelligent compromise you can derive enjoyment safely from other sports.

The level of skill you possess also may be an important consideration when you are trying to decide whether to return to a given sport. Snow sports are good examples. Skiers and ice skaters with years of experience and high degrees of skill can return to their activities much sooner than a novice should try such sports. Control to avoid injury, judgment to avoid excessive stress, and confidence to relax muscles that are not in active use allow the skilled to ski or to skate in spite of back conditions that would sideline the unskilled.

Most water sports are good recreation for people with back pain. Swimming may be quite beneficial. Water skiing is an exception. The very skilled may be able to control the dangers of water skiing, but the occasional skier is at risk of excessive back muscle strain, sudden twisting injuries, and the bouncing while twisting that so often occurs while riding in a ski boat.

Racket sports involve a lot of quick stop-and-go activity that can be stressful to the lower back. Handball requires more twisting stress to the lower back than sports in which you use rackets or paddles. Twisting and hyperextension of the back in tennis is most often associated with overhead shots and serving. When first trying to return to racket sports after a back injury, you will do best to begin with practice sessions of short duration using a backboard or with another player in a completely noncompetitive situation. Slowly increase the length of each workout and return to competitive playing and overhead shots only after you have demonstrated the ability to withstand long, noncompetitive workouts.

The same principles apply to such sports as basketball, softball, and soccer. Short practice sessions slowly working up to competitive intensity are necessary for a long while before you return to full effort. Such sports can be very vigorous contact sports or fairly relaxed fun activities, depending upon the competition and your attitude. You need to avoid approaching them with too much vigor until you are sure your back can take it. If you are too competitive to control those situations, you should stick with the fitness sports that carry less temptation to overdo.

Bowling probably causes more back problems to those with intermediate skills. There is little danger to those who are content to bend their knees enough, take a short approach, use a light ball, and forego a forceful twisting effort from a leaning position. For the very skilled, who have smooth deliveries and are always well balanced, there may be little risk of back injury. Those who are good enough to emulate the very skilled with a full run, full swing, and full force effort, but who lack perfect balance and timing, are in more danger of aggravating back pain. If you want to try bowling, you should exercise to simulate the bowling motion in the weeks before actual participation. Carefully warm up before each outing, and go easy the first few times.

Golf usually can be enjoyed by people with back pain. Short rounds and avoidance of full-effort, full-swing strokes are in order at first. The same smoothness, head and body control, and rhythmic movement that make for a good golf swing also provide safety for the back. The golfing motion that is most likely to be associated with pain is the twisting of the lower back during a full and forceful swing. You may find that the need to control and smooth your swing to avoid hurting your back actually improves your score, even if it shortens the distances of your longest drives. You need to apply the principles of car riding to golfcart riding.

Fishing, hunting, hiking, camping, and similar outdoor activities are subject to great variations in duration and intensity. Attention to the principles of good body mechanics and avoidance of stress beyond that to which you are accustomed allows safe return to these activities. Planning ahead so that you are certain not to be caught in situations where you must lift, carry, or accept other stresses beyond those for which you are conditioned is the most important consideration before return to these activities.

For recreation that involves riding, the duration must be tempered. Bumpy riding, such as horseback, trail bike, or jeep trail riding, may be quite stressful to the low back for people with disc disorders and should be approached cautiously. Speedboats may be dangerous because of the sudden forces with which you are bounced against the seat when slapping off waves. Even less stressful riding, such as in cars and road bikes, can produce back pain if the duration of the activity is too long at first. Most of these enjoyable activities can be pursued, even in the presence of back pain, if you use some caution about the vigor with which you go after them and follow the principles of good body mechanics.

One reason why many people forsake recreational activities when they have back pain is that they feel guilty about pursuing pleasure activity while they are avoiding responsibility at work or at home because of the pain. While your commitment to become well and to participate fully in life must include responsibilities, it should include fun, too.

Sometimes the fears that have built up can be dispelled by trying some of the fun things first. You should make a list of all of the things you have given up because of back pain. This should include both responsibilities that you feel you should do and fun things that you would like to do. Except for the things clearly out of bounds because of extreme back stress, you should work on that list, doing each of those things. Do them in moderation, but do them. Dispel the fear of trying, and get them off the list of things you can't do anymore because of back pain. If they cause you some pain the first time you try, don't give up—try a little smaller dose the next time. Chances are that the list has been getting longer and longer up until now. Now is the time to start making it smaller.

10
JOB FITNESS

U.S. Bureau of Labor statistics show that, in 1980, 1 million Americans sustained back injuries at work. Why did this happen? Don't people know how to do their jobs without getting hurt? Don't they physically condition themselves to withstand the stresses of their jobs? Are they not prepared to cope with the psychological stresses of their jobs and their lives? Might the figure be exaggerated because the American social structure provides incentives for workers to report back pains of unknown cause as work-related injuries? All of these possibilities are partially true. Each of those aspects of the problem is addressed elsewhere in this book. In this chapter, we will consider whether the jobs workers must do in industrialized nations may contribute to the high incidence of work-related back pain. We will also consider whether there might be better ways to match people with jobs they can do without injury.

Certain jobs statistically correlate with an increased incidence of back pain. There are, however, so many important things about individuals and particular job experiences that it is not valid to say that an individual's back pain is caused by the job, just because the job is one with a high incidence of back injury.

Injury may occur in three different ways. It helps to use the analogy of an automobile tire to distinguish these ways. There may be a sudden dramatic event that injures a perfectly sound back, like a new tire blowing out after rolling over a steel spike. There may be a less profound incident that brings the situation to notice, such as a tire weakened by wear and previous minor injury blowing out when it rolls over a rock. Finally, there may be no discernible event; the tire may have just gone flat because of too much wear and too many little, unnoticed bumps. This last concept may not seem like an injury at all, but it has been applied to certain back conditions considered to have resulted from cumulative trauma.

The type of injury that may have caused a particular back pain may have legal and economic importance. The different concepts of injury are also important to those who try to design jobs that will not cause back injury.

It takes a great deal of force to produce substantial injury to a normal human back. Most such injuries are the result of vehicle collision, falls from a height, or being struck by fallen material or heavy equipment. Prevention of such injuries has been the traditional role of occupational safety officers. In recent decades, the records of their achievements have been good. Though such injuries still occur and may be catastrophic, they do not explain the huge numbers and rising incidence of work-related back injuries.

Injuries that occur because of a relatively minor incident comprise the largest group of work-related back problems. Heavy lifting effort and slipping are reported with greatest frequency. The true correlation of back injury with a single episode of lifting or slipping is difficult to determine. There are incentives for workers to report the onset of their difficulty as related to such an incident and for doctors and lawyers to accept that report as valid. Workers often don't know exactly when the back pain started. They assume it was caused by a heavy effort or a slip that may have occurred at about that time. It is commonly accepted in our culture that back pain begins with such incidents, so it is reasonable for people to assume, if such an event occurred about the time when the pain started, that there was a causal relationship.

It may simplify assignments of legal responsibility to accept reports of lifting or slipping as causes of back injury. It may distort the picture, however, for those who are seeking ways to make jobs safer.

Whether or not we have a realistic picture of how often a single lifting effort is the sole cause of a back problem, there does seem to be a correlation between back trouble and jobs that require heavy lifting. At least, a larger percentage of workers who must do very heavy lifting report back injuries than those who do not do heavy lifting.

There are many ways to interpret the data that correlate back pain and heavy lifting, so it may not be wise to assume that any one individual is at greater risk because of a heavy lifting job. There are some data to suggest that a moderate frequency of heavy lifting, 50 to 150 efforts per week, is safer than either occasional or very frequent efforts.

Lifting objects from a stooped-over position, lifting objects out away from the body, lifting up to or down from overhead, and lifting while twisting all seem to correlate with back pain incidents. These correlations may apply both to isolated events of injury and as sources of repeated, minor traumas.

Recent studies from Great Britain and the United States provide evidence to suggest that back trouble may be related to vibration. Whole body vibration, such as that endured by truck drivers and heavy equipment operators, may occur at a frequency that is damaging to the spine. There is a lot more information needed before all of the reasons are understood, but there does seem to be a higher incidence of back injuries in occupations that involve whole body vibration. Whether segmental vibration, such as from operating vibrating tools, relates to back pain is less well known.

The idea of vibration as a cause of back injury depends upon acceptance of a controversial concept of cumulative trauma—that repeated minor stresses can lead eventually to harmful change. There is legal controversy about calling such a phenomenon an injury. There is also medical controversy. Some medical evidence and plausible theory supports the idea that cumulative trauma does cause harm. There is also theory and evidence to the contrary. An established principle of bone physiology, Wolfe's Law, is that bones get stronger when subjected to repeated stress—so, it seems, do the hearts of long-distance runners.

Young, strong, healthy people are less likely to hurt themselves by vigorous physical effort. Many years of the same stressful activity may lead to trouble in two ways. If the concept of cumulative trauma is valid, the years may produce an accumulation of harmful wear and tear. Also, the aging process diminishes resistance to injury. Either reason leads to the conclusion that careers should be designed so that those who must bear vigorous stress in their youth can graduate to less physically demanding work as they age.

Ideally, we should seek out correlations between specific occupational stresses and back injury and then eliminate those stresses by better job design. The study of work efficiency, design, and stress is called ergonomics. It is the job of those who work in ergonomics to seek the ideal so that jobs can be accomplished efficiently and without injury. They work the middle ground between medical research and industrial engineering.

The inadequacies of medical information and the demands of economic necessity make job safety through ergonomics a difficult task. When we make assumptions about the effects of various jobs on human anatomy, we jump huge gaps from observations of which activities seem to correlate with which jobs to minuscule knowledge about the anatomic changes that occur in response to such activities.

Even if job designers had complete, reliable medical information, economic factors would prevent them from fully applying it. Back injuries are serious problems, but so are unemployment and the economic survivals of industries and nations. To survive, employers must provide jobs, make a profit, sustain the economy, and keep their workers healthy. Those goals may be in conflict with one another. Elimination of the stresses that lead to back injury may help keep workers healthy but may also impair realization of the other goals and threaten the existence of the jobs.

Job Selection

If economic necessity requires that some jobs be done even if they have higher risks of back injury, it would be best to select people who are least apt to hurt their backs while doing those jobs. Another important way to look at that idea is that if you are seeking a job or a career, you should select what you are going to be able to sustain without injury.

Many employers have tried to include criteria that are predictive of back injury in their hiring practices. There are difficult problems in doing so. Statistical probability data cannot be applied to individual cases without charges of discrimination. The results have been hard to measure. An obvious consideration is age. A group of 50-year-olds will surely have more back injuries if assigned to lift 100-pound feedbags throughout the day than would a group of 20-year-olds. A well-conditioned 50-year-old with a good record at that kind of work may be at less risk than a poorly conditioned 20-year-old, however.

Sex discrimination related to back injury has been a volatile issue. Medical statistics about back injury look worse for men than for women, presumably because men have been more often in risky situations—an unproven presumption. Muscular strength protects against injury, and women generally are just 60 percent as strong as men—another generalization that may not apply to individuals. Pregnancies produce muscle and ligament changes that may impair resistance to back injuries.

There have been reports that tall people may suffer ruptured discs more frequently. Obese people may strain their backs more easily. People who have a previous history of back trouble, for a variety of reasons, are statistically more likely to have trouble again. So are those with a history of arthritis. And smokers have a higher incidence of back pain.

Preemployment x ray of the lumbar spine has been used widely.

Minor variations from normal have caused many people to be denied employment unjustly. There are x-ray abnormalities that may be found in certain individuals that would be just cause for them to avoid certain jobs. Such findings are so unusual that the indiscriminate use of pre-employment x rays is not justified.

Taking psychological histories and testing may help employers select those who are fit for certain jobs. People who abuse drugs or alcohol are more likely to have back injuries. Psychological testing for those who are highly anxious or depressed may be predictive of back injury risk, though there is no strong evidence that such is the case. Less conventional psychological testing to determine such things as motivation might come closer to the mark.

The problem with all of these selection criteria is that they are not really specific. They don't really test the individual's capacity to do the job. They only provide general information upon which a statistical bet can be made, and sometimes they don't even do that very well.

The obvious answer would be to test specifically for what the job would require. When the stress is periodic lifting effort, such testing may be feasible. When the worry is the effect of cumulative trauma over years of exposure, such testing is impractical.

Muscle strength testing would seem to be the way to determine the ability to do jobs that require forceful efforts. Indeed, it has been shown that if the maximum job load exceeds the average isometric strength of the individual, the injury risk is three times higher.

The theory behind muscle strength testing as a prerequisite to physically demanding jobs is good, but there are problems with design and application. The test must be safe. It must be reliable and quantitative so that fair comparisons can be made. It must test functions that relate to the specific job. It must be practical. Once all of those demands are met, it then must prove to be really predictive of injury risk.

Another obvious but often overlooked testing area is knowledge of technique. Applicants should be tested for their understanding of body mechanics as it relates to the job.

Selection processes, if they are valid at all, should apply to continuation at a given job. People should want to maintain the fitness level that is required for them to perform their job without injury.

Efforts by employers to exclude applicants from certain jobs on the basis of risk of back injury have been challenged in the courts. The Rehabilitation Act of 1973 covers hiring practices of U.S. projects. State laws vary. Generally, the employer, if challenged, must show that the decision was based upon a bona fide job requirement which was relevant to the applicant's failure to qualify or that the applicant's handicap would render him or her unable to perform the job without danger to his or her health or the health of others.

Individual Choices

Personal or economic need may mean that you must take some risks. Few people must exclude themselves absolutely from consideration of an occupation because of back trouble.

Your ability to perform certain jobs depends upon the effort you are willing to make and the risks you are willing to take. You must weigh the effort and the risks against your need and your opportunity. One-legged people have run marathons, deaf people have written symphonies, and people with serious back injuries have returned successfully to heavy manual labor and professional athletics. When they do, it requires acceptance of risks and extraordinary effort.

You may be excluded from certain things by doctor- or employer-imposed restrictions. Such restrictions are often reversible if you condition yourself and show determination to do the job.

Information about which jobs are dangerous to which people is fragmentary. It is hard to apply to individuals. It certainly shouldn't be the sole determinant of personal job decisions.

You must assess your physical and emotional strengths. You need to judge your current state of fitness, your potential fitness, and your motivation to maintain your potential. You need to evaluate your emotional, social, and economic needs as they relate to your work. You must look at the future of your work and at how you will be able to adapt your career to the physical limitations of aging. Weigh all of those factors, make the best decision for you, and then persist in your efforts to succeed.

11
EXERCISE

Almost everything you hear or read about back care advises some form of exercise. Yet some people feel that their back pain began in the first place because of exercise, that they have tried exercise and got no better or worse, or that exercise just seems impossible. To some, it seems contradictory to learn all the ways to keep from straining the back and then to be advised to exercise it. But there is a great deal of misunderstanding about what is meant by exercise and how it applies to low back problems. Once you understand it, it is apparent how important exercise is to a healthy back.

Some exercises can produce stresses that could cause the back to hurt, maybe even the same stresses that led to the back problem in the first place. The differences between accepting these stresses in the form of exercise and allowing them to occur at other times is that, with exercise, stress is monitored and controlled. By slowly building up to and beyond the point where injury might have occurred, you make the supporting structures ready to accept the stress without ill effect.

The need to avoid excess stress, as taught in Chapters 2 and 3, and the need to develop tolerance to stress, as taught in this chapter, are not contradictory. The two needs must be balanced and coordinated. Both techniques must be learned and applied together as best suits you at the time. What posture and mechanical stresses are acceptable and what exercise level is desirable change all the time—with proper application, they change in the direction that provides better function and less pain.

The most common complaint about exercises made by back pain sufferers is that they tried it and it didn't help. In almost every case, the effort was too brief. Usually, the purpose and the techniques of the exercises are not well understood. Often, initial enthusiasm leads to efforts that are too vigorous, and the pain that results leads to discouragement. Exercises done properly will help almost everyone. It takes dedication and patience, but the rewards are plentiful.

There are, of course, many different types of exercise. An almost endless variety of activities can be termed exercise. Exercises may be divided into a small number of groups, depending on the goal of the exercise. We will consider five groups: exercises done for posture, those done for relaxation, those that promote motion and flexibility, those that build strength, and those that produce general fitness. Coordination, another goal of exercise, is obtained from combinations of flexibility and general fitness exercises and recreational activity.

Many exercises lead toward more than one of these goals. Each person will have different goals and will have different capabilities to use the exercises that help achieve those goals. Exercise prescriptions are not the same for everyone. Exercise programs and goals do not always remain the same for the same people. By understanding the goals and the principles of the exercises that lead to their achievement, you will be able to choose what will be safest, most effective, and most pleasant for you. Then, as you progress, you will be able to adjust your exercise program to tailor it to your needs.

Exercise for Posture

Poor posture habits may result from weak muscles, tight muscles or joints, psychological problems, being overweight, habit, ignorance of good posture, and, most often, a combination of those factors. Correction of poor posture habits, regardless of their cause, can improve or prevent back pain. The correction will be aided by direct attack on underlying problems by strengthening weak muscles and stretching tight muscles. In this section, however, we will consider some shortcut exercises that go directly to the posture problem.

The pelvic tilt is a basic exercise of most back care programs. In itself, it is a good posture exercise. It serves as a starting point for other exercises and for the performance of many strenuous activities, so it is a good exercise to learn and apply first. To begin, do a supine pelvic tilt from a lying-down, face-up position. Bend your knees and put your feet flat. Place your hand flat in the arch of your low back and feel the space between your low back and the floor, the space created because of your lumbar lordosis. Now remove your hand and relax your arms at your side. Tighten your buttock muscles together as though trying to hold a coin between them. Now tighten your abdominal muscles so that the arch of your lower back disappears and you reduce your lordosis. You should feel your stomach suck in and your pelvic bone tilt upward. Once you get the feel of this, progress to where you actually lift your buttocks up an inch or two from the surface. Do not, however, allow your back to come up from the floor.

Now do a standing pelvic tilt. (See Figure 7.) Stand with your back to a wall so your hips, heels, and shoulders touch the wall. Reach your hand in to feel the space between your low back and the wall. Now remove your hand, suck in your stomach, tighten your buttock muscles, tilt your pelvis, and reduce your lordosis. Once you can do this successfully, you will no longer be able to slide your hand between your lower back and the wall. Feel yourself get taller by straightening your back. The pelvic tilt is basic to proper standing and walking posture and especially as a preparation to any sudden exertion such as lifting or carrying.

One way to practice "getting tall" is to imagine that there is a wire attached to the middle of the top of your head. Imagine a gentle but firm upward pull so that the weight of your upper body is overcome, your neck is pulled up straight and in line with your back, your pelvis swings forward, and your lower back straightens. Once you get this help to get

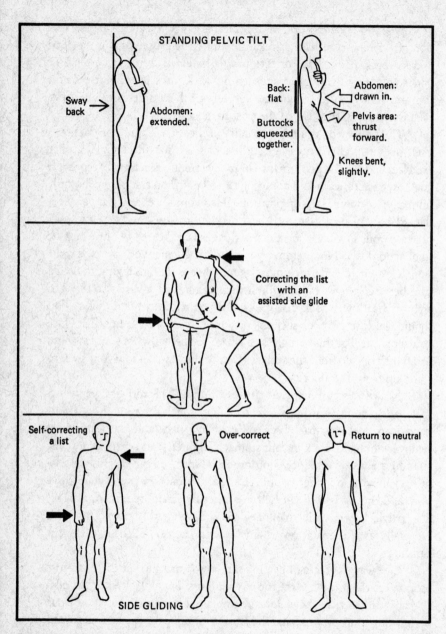

FIGURE 7. Posture Exercises.

you tall, then you can relax a little—let your jaw loosen so your teeth are not touching, let your shoulders drop down (but not forward), and breathe deeply and easily.

Another posture problem that is common to many people with back pain is a tendency to stand tilted to one side. Sometimes this is the result of permanent structural change in the lower back or because of muscle pull away from a position that would cause pain. More often, it is a result of muscles or ligaments that have become tight in that position after the need to avoid pain has passed. Sometimes it simply results from habit. This tendency to lean to one side is called a list. Some people tend always to list to the same side, and others may list to the right at one time and to the left another time.

The posture exercise used to correct a list is called side gliding. (See Figure 7.) First, stand with your feet comfortably spaced and your weight balanced so your hips are level. Then shift or glide your upper body away from the side of the list. You may do the lateral bending exercise, which you will read about under the description of flexibility exercises, to loosen up, but it is not the same. The difference is that with the side glide your shoulders stay level and you make no attempt to slide your hand down the side of your thigh.

When you first learn side gliding, it may help to have someone push your pelvis toward the side of the list and at the same time push your chest and shoulders to the opposite side. That way, you can get the feel of the gliding movement while you concentrate on keeping your head, shoulders, and pelvis level. Try to overcorrect the list so that you lean in the opposite direction and then come back to the neutral, straight-up position. Repeat the exercise often throughout the day until you overcome the tendency to list.

The stresses from sitting are quite different from those of standing and lying, and they require different practices and exercises. The method to obtain the correct sitting posture was described in Chapter 2. You should use that method as a posture exercise if you spend much of your day sitting. If you sit for more than an hour at a time, you should stand, place your hands on your buttocks, tilt your head and shoulders back, and arch your back into full extension a few times at least every hour. The same applies if you work bending forward from a standing position.

Once you master the feelings of tilting your pelvis, getting tall, side gliding, and doing sitting posture exercises, you do not always have to be doing your exercises to practice these techniques. They are easy, low-energy activities that can be done over and over throughout the day without fear of exhaustion or of overworking the muscles. Make a habit of doing them at idle moments, in response to twinges of back pain, or in preparation for any stressful activity.

Relaxation Exercises

Most people feel the tensions that build up as a result of the demands and frustrations of life. Tensions aren't always felt in the same way. Sometimes they may be felt as headache, sometimes as nervousness, sometimes as fatigue, and sometimes as back pain. Often, the result is muscle tenseness.

Muscle tension may build gradually without you being aware of its presence. By the time tension causes pain, it may have been present a long while and may be pretty severe. Then the pain it causes is one more frustration that leads to more tension, more pain, and on it goes.

Back pain is a frequent component of this cycle. Sometimes tension is the most important factor in back pain. Almost always, it is at least some portion of the problem. Even pains caused by such obviously explainable things as broken bones or operations are made much worse by tension.

One way to interrupt the tension–pain–tension cycle is to learn to recognize and control some of the frustrations that lead to tension. That approach is discussed in Chapter 5.

Another approach is to recognize the muscle tension when it starts to build and to apply techniques to relax the muscles before the tension begins to make the pain worse.

Some people object to calling relaxation techniques exercise. They fear that just the mention of exercise may cause tension and make relaxation difficult. One of the things you want, however, is to dispel any notions you have that exercise is unpleasant. Different forms of exercise produce feelings of well-being and relaxation in different ways and at different times. Fitness and strengthening exercises, done properly, leave you with those feelings afterward. Relaxation exercises are meant to help you achieve those feelings directly, during the exercise period, ideally with a carryover effect into the rest of the day.

Like the posture exercises, relaxation exercises can be done as often as you wish without fear of overdoing it. They should be done at times when you feel the tension building, at times and in situations when you have observed tension building, and when you want to be fully relaxed, such as before you begin stretching and strengthening exercises.

It may help to perform a little experiment to demonstrate the effects of tension. Stand with your back flat against the wall, then move your feet out about one step, bend your knees, and lower your buttocks a little more than halfway down to sitting posture. See how long you can stay there. The answer will depend on your state of conditioning, how far you bend your knees, and your pain tolerance, but it won't be long. The pain you feel in the big muscles in front of your thighs is the result of sustained muscle tension. It's not hard to understand how the muscles of the back cause pain if, for whatever reason, they are maintained in a tense state for long.

Many different techniques or exercises are designed to achieve relaxation. Variations on commonly used ones are presented here as examples. Most people can employ these techniques effectively on their own. The use of tapes, equipment such as biofeedback devices, and professional guidance (such as from a psychological, occupational, or physical therapist) can increase the proficiency with which these methods are used and are recommended for those who cannot achieve the desired result on their own.

The contrast relaxation exercise is not only an effective tool to achieve relaxation but is also another demonstration of the feel of muscle tension.

Contrast Relaxation Exercises. Use a quiet room away from phone, television, radio, or other distractions. A tape to guide you through the exercise or soft instrumental music may be played, but otherwise silence is best. Dim the lights, loosen tight clothing, and remove tight or heavy jewelry. Lie in the rest position on a rug or exercise mat. Take three deep, easy breaths. You are going to alternately tighten and relax various muscles. By doing so, you will learn the feeling of tension and the feeling of relaxation. Tighten muscles gradually at first. Do not make them hurt. Continue to breathe deeply and easily throughout the exercise.

Tighten the right hand into a fist. Hold for five seconds, thinking, "My hand is tense." Then let go and let the fingers fall loose and limp. Think, "My fingers are warm and relaxed." Do this three times; then repeat with the left hand three times.

Now raise the right arm up, clench the fist, bend the elbow by forcing the fist to the shoulder, and tighten all of the shoulder and neck muscles. Hold for five seconds, thinking, "My arm is tense." Then let the arm flop down. Think, "My arm is heavy, warm, and relaxed." After three times with the right arm, do the same thing three times with the left arm.

Move the ankles, heels, and knees together so that they touch each other. Now squeeze them as tightly together as you can. Start with the ankles. Then, keeping the ankles tight, force the knees tightly together. Keep knees and ankles tightly squeezed together; then tighten the buttock muscles together. Hold everything tight for five seconds, thinking, "My legs are tense." Then suddenly relax all of the muscles. Feel the heaviness of your legs and your hips against the floor. Think, "My legs are heavy, warm, and relaxed." Now shrug your shoulders up to your ears. Press your shoulder blades and upper back down, hard against the floor. Think, "My back is tense." Hold for five seconds. Then let it all go and feel your back and shoulders sink. Think, "My back is heavy, warm, and relaxed."

Push the back of your head down tightly against the floor. Tense the neck muscles in front and back, clenching the teeth. Think, "My neck is tense." Now relax. Feel your head heavy against the floor. Feel the heaviness of your jaw as it drops open and your teeth separate. Tell yourself, "My head is heavy, warm, and relaxed." Pucker up your lips very tightly and hold for three seconds; then relax and let the lips go slack. Then pull the mouth into a deep frown. Hold for three seconds, feeling the tension; then let go. Smile broadly for three seconds; then let go. Wrinkle up the nose for three seconds; then let it relax. Raise the eyebrows and tense the wrinkles in the forehead for three seconds; then let them go and let the forehead smooth. Squint the eyes tightly shut. Hold them for three seconds; then relax, letting the lids droop almost closed. Now tense all of the face muscles together and hold for five seconds. Then relax. Feel your forehead go smooth and all tension leave your face. Repeat this three times.

Now lie quietly, limp and free. Feel the heaviness of your arms, legs, and head and the smoothness of your face. Breathe easily and deeply, saying to yourself with each breath, "Relax." Learn this feeling of being relaxed so you can recall it anytime during your day.

This series of exercises and others using the same principles are called contrast relaxation exercises. By consciously tensing the muscles so you can really feel them tense, you can become aware of that tense feeling and then can contrast that with the relaxation that follows. The same principle can be used to obtain relaxation in various situations throughout the day without having to interrupt for an exercise session.

Meditation. Meditation is often associated with mystical, spiritual, or exotic practices. These associations are not necessarily valid. Unless combined with spiritual or mystical elements, meditation is a simple, healthful practice, unusual only in its contrast to the pace of the rest of contemporary society.

The purpose of meditation is to calm the mind by limiting attention to a single focus. This may involve chanting a word or focusing on a spiritual image, but when meditating for practical, healthful purposes, you usually can focus on the breath. All of the mind's chatter and static of worries, plans, and fantasies are regarded as intrusions on the process of concentrating on this one subject—the breath. Any other neutral, always available subject or image can be chosen if you have any reason to prefer it to the breath.

Meditation is a skill to be learned by practice. Devotion of time and effort are required. Until mastered, meditation should be practiced at least daily, preferably at the same time and in the same place. Allow 20 minutes. Make every effort to secure freedom from interruptions and intruding noises. Use a timer so you know when the time is up without having to check periodically. Begin with an alert mind. Don't practice meditation at a time when you are usually sleepy. You can meditate recumbent or seated in the classic lotus position, but for most novices meditation is done best when seated in a straight chair with a comfortably padded but hard seat.

Sit so that the front edge of the chair strikes you at midthigh. The height of the chair should be such that the knees are at about hip height. Have both feet flat on the floor so that the angle between the lower legs and thighs is a little more than 90 degrees. Let the arms hang limp at the side and hold the lower back comfortably straight. Rock back and forth a little until you find a neutral, balanced position. Next, allow your head to roll about over your shoulders a little until it, too, finds a neutral position over the shoulders. Now lift your hands and allow them to flop across your inner thighs so that the weight of your forearms comes to rest on your thighs.

This neutral, balanced posture can be used as a starting point for contrast relaxation exercises, deep relaxation, or meditation. Close your eyes and pay attention to your breathing. Follow each breath all the way in and all the way out. Think only of the breathing. If any other thought comes to mind, allow it to pass right on through. Every other thought should be only a reminder to return your concentration to the breathing.

You may wish to count the breaths. Count up to ten and then start over. You may want to incorporate some word or image into the counting. This may allow you to recall the word in times of stress and, with it, to recall some of the feelings of serenity you experienced while meditating.

You also may use the image of some surrounding color, usually a restful color such as blue or green. You may image your tension as a harsh color and then think of drops falling into it, fading it, and then converting it to a restful color.

Whether you count, use a word or phrase in rhythm, or use some visual image with the breathing, such techniques should only complement your attention to the breathing. No thoughts of productivity or obligation, no worries, no longings or regrets are to intrude on this concentration on breathing. Every such thought reminds you to think only of the breathing and then passes right on by.

When you have completed your meditation time, open your eyes. Look at and sense your body. Note how relaxed you are. Stretch and arise alert and relaxed.

Those who meditate regularly do so because they feel less stress and are able to maintain tension-free alertness more successfully when they do so. The benefits are more apparent after weeks of practice. It is often difficult at first to concentrate and achieve full benefit from the technique. Once mastered, however, meditation may be recalled, like typing or riding a bicycle, more easily than it was first learned.

Deep Relaxation. Another deep relaxation technique involves some elements of both the contrast relaxation and meditation. This technique is more complex, so it is best for you to have an assistant read the instructions or to use a tape until you master the technique. You may start in various positions, and the instructions vary depending on the position. To provide something different from the back-lying rest position, the following instruction for this type of exercise is given for lying on the right side on a bed. The floor or an exercise mat also can be used.

You should be in a quiet, dimly lit room. All outside thoughts and worries should pass right through without your thinking about them. Be sure that you will not be interrupted. Lie on your right side with a small, soft pillow under the right side of your head. Both legs are bent at the knee. The left leg is pulled up higher toward the chest and rests on a pillow in front of the right leg. The right arm is behind the back with the elbow bent comfortably, the back of the hand against the bed, and the fingers open. The left arm is in front with the hand palm-down at face level.

Feel the heaviness of your body against the bed. Feel that heaviness sink your body down into the bed. Don't be afraid. Let it go heavier and heavier, deeper and deeper. Don't force it; just let it happen. Feel your weight pull down. Feel your eyes loose and heavy. Your forehead is smooth and wide. Your lips are limp. Your teeth are apart. Push your tongue hard against the roof of your mouth, harder and harder. Feel it tense your face muscles, even down into your neck and chest. Now let your tongue fall, heavy and limp, down against the teeth on the right side of your mouth. Feel how heavy your tongue is. Feel how relaxed your face and head are.

Let yourself be more relaxed than before. You are heavier, sinking deeper. Now feel where the right foot touches the bed. Feel the contact. Feel the heaviness. Feel the pull, the binding between the foot and the bed. Feel the foot sink into the bed; become part of it. Now feel the right knee and everywhere that touches between the foot and the knee. Feel the leg and floor pull together. Feel the leg flow into the bed and become part of it. Now feel the right hip. Feel the heaviness of the pelvis pushing down and the hip flowing and sinking into the bed. Feel the upper leg. Feel where the foot touches the bed. Feel it flow into the bed, sinking down and becoming part of it. Feel the heaviness all along the left leg as it flows into the pillow. Everywhere the leg touches, it sinks down in. Feel the heaviness of the left hip and the thigh as it sinks down in. As the hip and thigh become more limp and heavier, they push the right side further down, making it heavier and sinking it deeper into the bed.

Now feel all along the side and the chest. Feel the heaviness; feel the pull down into the bed. Feel the muscles let go under the collarbone. The left side of the chest is loose and heavy and falls down against the right side, which is sinking heavier into the bed. Feel the right shoulder being pulled down where it touches—sinking, binding, becoming part of the bed. Feel the same heaviness all along the right arm where it lies against the bed. The arm is heavy, pulled down into the bed. Feel the back of the hand heavy, sinking down, flowing into the bed where it touches. Feel the fingers open and loose. Feel the blood flow through the fingertips, making them warm and relaxed. The left shoulder is heavy, loose, sinking down, pushing the right shoulder down deeper. The left arm, all along where it touches the bed, becomes heavier and heavier. The arm is sinking in. The left hand is heavy, the palm sinking in, becoming part of the bed. The fingertips are warm where they touch. The blood flowing in them warms them, and the warmness flows into the bed.

Your head is very heavy, sinking down into the pillow. It is pulled down, flowing into the pillow. You let it go. You feel your head let go under your ears, behind the base of your skull. You are not afraid. You allow yourself to sink deeper. Your cheeks and lips sag. Your tongue is heavy, drooping against the side of your teeth. Your eyelids are heavy. Your forehead is smooth. You sink deeper and deeper. You are not afraid. You are completely relaxed. Remain that way for a moment and then stretch and arise, refreshed and relaxed.

Keep Tension in Balance. Few people can spend their lives meditating and devoting full attention to relaxation. Everyone, though, needs some break from the tensions of life. Many things that bring on tensions are also pleasurable and profitable—spouse, kids, jobs—so you can't always avoid them. If you learn these relaxation techniques, you will have ways to give your muscles a break from tension.

Strengthening Exercises

Stronger muscles are more resistant to injury. Strong muscles are more able to protect the underlying bones and ligaments from injury. Increased strength means better tone and improved ability to maintain correct posture.

Strengthening exercises do not have to be done as often as flexibility exercises. You should do a full set of strengthening exercises every other day. At each session, make at least ten efforts at each exercise. Each effort should last from two to five seconds. If you cannot do the full range of the exercise, a determined effort is what counts. Once you can accomplish the full range ten times, you may progress by adding more repetitions, or you may switch to a more difficult exercise for the same muscles.

Abdominal Muscle Strengthening. The lower back obtains primary muscular support from groups of muscles that connect the spine to the ribs and pelvis. The muscles of the abdomen are large muscles that have the potential to lend considerable support to the low back. When you hold the abdominal contents firmly, they exert a hydrostatic pressure over the whole front of the spine. Because the abdominal muscles connect your ribs to the front of your pelvis, they help prevent your low back from sagging into lordosis.

The lumbar spine and the abdominal contents are encased within a cylinder of large muscles. Cylindrical structures lose strength if a weak spot is created in them. Invert a paper cup and push down evenly on it, testing its resistance to collapse. Then tear a nickle-size hole out of the side and repeat the test. The strength of any one point on the cylinder depends on the whole cylinder being intact.

Unfortunately, several things may weaken abdominal muscles, depriving them of their ability to support the spine. Pregnancy, abdominal surgery, and obesity are common causes of abdominal muscle weakness. Often, inadequate exercise of the abdominal muscles leads to the trouble. Combinations of these factors are responsible for a lot of back pain.

Abdominal muscles stretched out by pregnancies or by too much abdominal fat lose their tone. Regaining the strength and tone requires a lot of effort over a long time. Sometimes the exercises needed to build back the abdominal muscles may cause some pain. However, the alternative of letting the muscles get weaker and weaker, allowing the abdomen to protrude and the back to sag, can only lead to greater trouble.

The situp is the best exercise for strengthening abdominal muscles. (See Figure 8.) Full flexion of the lumbar spine against a tight abdomen is too much back stress for beginners and for those in pain. The benefits can be achieved without coming all the way up.

Lie on your back with knees bent and feet flat on the floor. By keeping your knees bent, you keep tension off your sciatic nerve. You also neutralize your hip flexor muscles so you must make the full effort with your abdominal muscles. Your arms should lie comfortably at your sides. Breathing is relaxed and normal. Pull smoothly up until your head and shoulders are off the surface. Feel the strain in the abdominal muscles. Hold the position, breathing normally for a second or two at first. Gradually increase the time you hold the position and the number of repetitions.

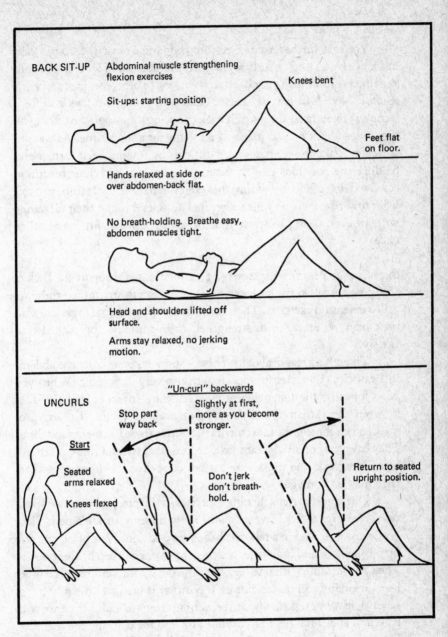

FIGURE 8. Situps and Uncurls.

You may further strengthen your abdominal muscles through their full range by adding uncurls to the partial situps. (See Figure 8.) Start in a sitting position with your back straight, knees bent, feet flat, and arms relaxed. Now lean partway back. Hold your trunk and legs still for a second or two; then pull yourself back to sitting up straight. At first, you should lean back only a little way and only for a short time. As you get stronger, make the exercise more difficult by leaning back further and holding the positions longer. Keep your feet flat and your breathing easy, and don't jerk. By adding this exercise to the partial situp, you can work toward exercising your abdominal muscles through their full range without ever having to stress your back through that full range all at once.

Back Extensor Muscle Strengthening. The muscles that support the back of the spine are called the back extensors. Exercises to strengthen them are called extension exercises. These muscles are apt to be sore in people with back pain, so exercises to strengthen them must be approached cautiously.

Though a great deal of lower back support comes from the abdominal muscles, the extensor muscles are also very important. When you bend forward, the ligaments of your back are stretched and the discs between the vertebrae in front are put under pressure. The extensor muscles can control the movements that stress those ligaments and discs. They have the potential to absorb a great deal of stress if they are strong. If they are weak, the stresses are passed to the discs and ligaments where they may do damage.

Do extensor strengthening exercises in the prone (face-down) position. (See Figure 9.) Have a small pillow under your abdomen. Place both arms overhead in a relaxed, hands-up position. First bring one arm up off the floor and hold it for a second or two, and then bring it down. Then do the same with one leg, then the other arm, and then the other leg. Gradually add on seconds each position is held and the number of repetitions. Progress slowly. After gaining strength and confidence with one limb at a time, begin to lift one arm and the opposite leg together. Later, begin with both arms together and both legs together. Progress to

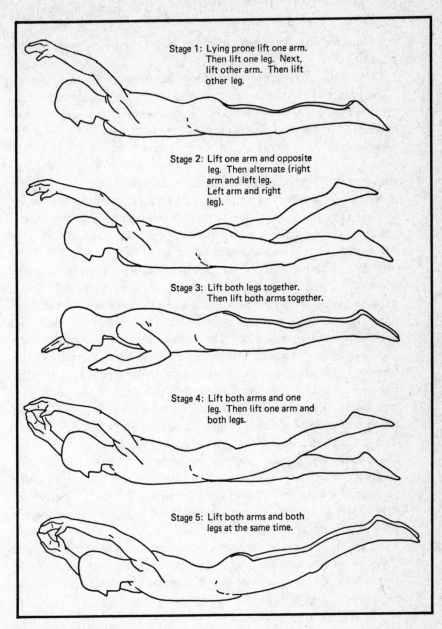

Stage 1: Lying prone lift one arm. Then lift one leg. Next, lift other arm. Then lift other leg.

Stage 2: Lift one arm and opposite leg. Then alternate (right arm and left leg. Left arm and right leg).

Stage 3: Lift both legs together. Then lift both arms together.

Stage 4: Lift both arms and one leg. Then lift one arm and both legs.

Stage 5: Lift both arms and both legs at the same time.

FIGURE 9. Back Extension Exercises.

three limbs at once and finally to lifting both arms and both legs at the same time.

As with all exercises, these progressions must be taken slowly. Many people have increased pain when doing situps or extension exercises. Almost always, the reason is that the attempts at progress are too rapid. Adding on more repetitions or more difficult exercises should be done in small increments and at weekly—not daily—intervals.

Hip and Thigh Strengthening. Strong hip and thigh muscles support your lower back by stabilizing your pelvis and providing steady support to the legs. The rhythm and strength of the hip and leg muscles allow expert tennis players, golfers, karate performers, and other athletes to exert tremendous body forces without back injury.

Wall slide exercises are an excellent beginning for hip extensor and quadriceps (front of the thigh) strengthening. (See Figure 10.) Stand with your back flat against a wall, feet 12 inches out from the wall, and pelvis tilted. Bend your knees and slide down the wall. Hold the position, breathing normally. Then push your knees straight and slide back up. Bending your knees more adds more stress. Start out by bending as far as you can for five seconds with ten repetitions. Increase the degree of the bend, the duration of the hold, and the number of repetitions as you become stronger. To avoid knee injuries, do not progress beyond 60 degrees of knee flexion.

Another excellent way to gain thigh and hip muscle strength is to ride a stationary bicycle. Keep the seat up high to avoid excessive knee bending, and adjust the handle bars to a position that is comfortable for your back. People with certain back conditions (stenosis, for example) may be able to exercise more effectively in the seated, slightly forward-leaning position of the bicyclist.

The muscles of the side of the hip (abductors) may be strengthened if you lie on your side and lift your leg up. Hold for a second or two at first. Don't jerk or hold your breath. Gradually increase the time you hold your leg up and the number of repetitions.

Upper Extremity Strengthening Exercises. Strong arm and shoulder muscles allow you to make vigorous efforts with lifting, pushing, and pulling

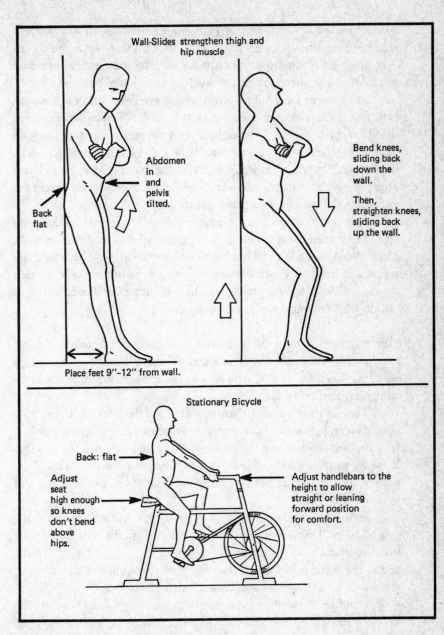

FIGURE 10. Leg Strengthening Exercises.

without having to transfer the stress to your lower back. If your work or recreation requires vigorous physical effort with your arms and shoulders, you need to condition your upper extremity muscles. Failure to do so places you at increased risk of hurting your lower back.

Most upper extremity strengthening exercises can be done with little fear of aggravating back pain if you follow the principles of caution that have been repeated throughout this chapter. You should avoid particularly exercises that force your back into excessive lordosis under the stress of weight. Overhead weight lifting, as when doing a military press, weighted squats, and standing curls, may produce excessive lordosis if the weight is not well controlled.

If you lift weights to strengthen your upper extremities, you should take some extra precautions to protect your back. Wear a weight lifter's belt or an abdominal binder. Do exercises with your back partially supported, such as bench presses and standing curls with your back against a wall. Always limit the weight and number of lifts to what you can do while maintaining good back posture.

Swimming Pool Exercises. Many exercises can be done efficiently and, for some people, more pleasantly in water. Those with regular access to a pool may use it for general fitness exercises and also for some strengthening and flexibility exercises.

The elementary back stroke provides good shoulder and upper back strengthening exercise. Pull your arms through the water to shoulder level and then back to your sides. Use either a frog style or a flutter kick. It is easy to avoid excessive lumbar lordosis in this position. This is the swimming stroke that can be done with least stress to the bones and joints of the spine.

Pool exercises should be done in chest-high water. Hold on to the side of the pool with your arms. With your back to the wall, bring your knees to your chest; then straighten your legs with your hips at a right angle. Force the legs apart against the water resistance. Rest a second; then force them together and cross them like scissors.

Stand and raise one leg at a time with your knee bent; then force the knee out straight, pause, and then forcefully bring the leg down against the water resistance.

With your side to the wall, kick your leg forcefully out to the side, pause, and then forcefully bring it back in. Face the wall and kick the leg forcefully back, keeping the knee straight. Pause, and bring it forcefully back down. Hold on to the side with your back to the wall and bicycle kick.

As with all exercises, there is no one correct number of repetitions or duration of effort for pool exercises. Begin easily and slowly progress to gain strength.

Building Slowly. Remember that building muscle strength takes time. The stresses that put tough calluses on the palms by repeated, gradual, increasing effort will cause painful blisters if done too rapidly. Strength and fitness require lifetime commitment. There is nothing to be gained by trying to hurry the progress beyond that for which you are prepared.

Flexibility Exercises

Stiffness may result from limited joint motion, limited ability of the muscles and tendons to stretch, or both. Lack of exercise and tension are the major culprits that lead to stiffness.

Stretching beyond the limits of easy motion usually involves some discomfort. Even perfectly healthy people who have never had anything wrong with their backs or joints have pain when stressed beyond that to which they are accustomed. Any healthy person trying to do a split for the first time certainly would experience pain, and if the split were accomplished, probably would experience serious injury. Very few people are born able to do a split. Most of those who can do so became able by patient, careful, repeated effort.

The same patient, careful, repeated effort that enables people to learn to move joints beyond what is normal can bring back lost normal motion.

Stiff muscles and joints hurt when stretched even within the usual or normal range. That is one good reason to exercise—to try to gain flexibility and eliminate stiffness. There is more reason than that, however. Loss of normal motion prevents normal posture. Muscles and joints work together so that loss of normal motion in one muscle may result in loss of some motion in the joint it crosses. This, in turn, causes other joints to position themselves abnormally. If the muscles or ligaments across the front of your hip are stiff, for example, your thigh won't come down straight from your pelvis when your pelvis is in a normal standing position. You have to stand with your hip flexed a little; and when you do, you must sway your lower back into lordosis so your upper body will be upright.

Even a stiff ankle can cause such problems. If your heel cord and calf muscles are tight, they will tend to pitch you forward a little. Unless there is enough extra motion in your hips and knees to make up for that, you will stand upright at the expense of your lower back. High-heeled shoes may cause a similar problem.

Caution, Timing, and Patience. Motion is lost because of prolonged tension, too little exercise, poor posture, and, in some instances, disorders of the underlying anatomy. These changes almost always occur slowly. Even if the symptoms began abruptly, the changes that cause persisting stiffness occur over a long time. You cannot reverse those changes rapidly. It takes time and a lot of patience and persistence to regain motion.

Many people are stiff in the early mornings. It may help to do gentle flexibility exercises before getting out of bed. Accept, though, that you may not have the range of free motion then that you will have later in the day, so expect a little less and don't hurt yourself. The discs are a little swollen in the mornings, so rapid, jerking, twisting movements should be avoided during the morning flexibility exercises. It is best to do your most vigorous flexibility exercises later in the day.

It may be easier to stretch more motion into stiff, sore muscles if you first apply heat to the affected areas. Warm clothing also helps.

Before doing any exercise to stretch tight structures, it is best to warm up with a simple relaxing motion. The rocking exercise works well as a warmup for people with back pain. Lie on the bed or on the floor on your back. Bend your knees and put the soles of your feet together. Now, gently and rhythmically, rock your body from side to side. From the same position, tilt your pelvis up and down a few times. Then proceed to flexibility exercises.

The number of repetitions of any one exercise and the number of sessions that you work on the exercise each day will vary with your needs and abilities. After you try out the exercises, you may apply the following guidelines to determine what schedule will be best for you.

If you lack flexibility in certain muscles or joints, it will be necessary to do very frequent exercises to regain the lost motion. Exercise daily or every other day may be adequate for general fitness and strengthening, but it will not be satisfactory for regaining lost motion. You should have one or two sessions every day in which you make a vigorous, concentrated effort to push new motion into the stiff area. You should supplement that with frequent but more gentle repetitions of the exercise throughout the day. Do ten repetitions of the exercise every waking hour or two. It may be necessary to continue at this frequency for two months or more in order to maintain early progress.

After your most vigorous flexibility exercise session, it may help to apply ice for 20 minutes to areas that have been sore. Ice packs help whenever you think you may have injured yourself by overstretching.

You may have to endure some discomfort in order to regain motion in stiff backs and joints. Forceful efforts to regain motion rapidly can be outright painful and should be avoided. Excessive force could even be dangerous if you have bones weakened by osteoporosis or a disc about to rupture. If you learn proper techniques and are patient with your progress, you are not likely to harm yourself.

Active and Passive Exercises. Several types of exercises may help with flexibility. Passive exercises are done to you by someone else with no effort on your part except to relax. Passive exercise has the disadvantage of requiring the presence of someone else. That person must be helpful but gentle and must understand that sudden jerking, forceful motions are not helpful and could be harmful.

Exercises done purely on your own are called active exercises. A purely active exercise involves only the use of your own muscles to exert the force.

Many exercises combine active and passive elements. You can use gravity to assist your active effort by positioning yourself so that some of your body weight exerts part of the force. This is a form of active assisted exercise.

When help is available, another form of active assisted exercise may be done. The basic effort comes from active muscle push, but a little extra push or an assist in holding what has been gained is added by an assistant.

Back and Leg Motions. Your lower back bends in three different planes. The greatest motion is in flexion and extension as when bending forward to touch your toes and arching back to look at the ceiling. The lower back bends from side to side when you reach your fingers straight down the side of your leg to the side of your knee—a motion called lateral bending If you stand with your hips still and turn your head and shoulders as though to look behind you, motion occurs in the third plane—rotation. Most ordinary movements of the back involve combinations of motion in these three planes.

Motion in the hip occurs in the same three planes. The greatest motion is in flexion as when you bend your knee toward your chest. The opposite motion in the same plane—extension—normally occurs to a little beyond the straight position.

The arc of normal hip flexion and extension permits most of the flexibility of the pelvic area. In fact, most of what is usually thought of as bending the back to pick up something from the floor is actually bending of the hip. Most ordinary activities of that sort can be accomplished by people with stiff, painless backs, if their hip motion is normal. The entire lumbar spine will only flex about 45 degrees, whereas normal hips will bend at least 120 degrees.

Side-to-side motion at the hip is called abduction and adduction. Abduction is the motion of the hip required to spread the legs apart. Adduction is the opposite motion used to close or cross the legs. You can feel hip rotation movement if you lie flat and turn your foot inward to a pigeon-toed position and then outward so the toes of each foot point away from each other.

The normal knee moves very slightly in rotation and from side to side. The only knee motion that occurs through enough range to be important to back problems is that of flexion and extension. The same is true of the ankle joint.

The joints of the foot must allow the foot to conform to the walking and standing surface. Under unusual circumstances, stiffness in these joints may contribute to back pain.

Back Flexibility Exercises. Flexion (forward bending) and extension (backward bending) of the lumbar spine are done in the same plane of motion. Some exercises push to the limit in both directions. You want full motion in both directions, but it is likely that you have more stiffness, more pain, and more need for work with one direction than the other. You also may have some reason to limit one direction or the other. You may want, therefore, to use one of the more advanced flexion–extension exercises to gain motion in one direction while using a beginning exercise for the other direction.

You may do exercises to gain flexion from a supine (lying face-up) posture. (See Figure 11.) Pull one knee at a time up to the chest as a preliminary stretch. This single knee-chest lift is an excellent exercise to improve hip motion. To get your lower back to bend into flexion, you pull both knees toward your chest at the same time—the double knee-to-chest lift. Keep your back flat as your legs come up; then feel your back flex as your pelvis and shoulders roll forward. Pull with your hands under your thighs and let your knees bend comfortably.

You may do extension exercises in the prone (lying face-down) position. Prop your upper body on your elbows as a preliminary stretch. Keep the pelvis down. Progress to doing pushoffs by pushing your upper body up while leaving your pelvis and lower body down flat. It may help to have someone hold your hips down. After you stretch out the tight structures in the front of your lumbar spine and hips, however, you should be able to do this unassisted.

Flexion and extension flexibility exercises can be done from the hands-and-knees position. Let your back sag into lordosis as much as you can; then reverse the position and arch the lower back up like an angry

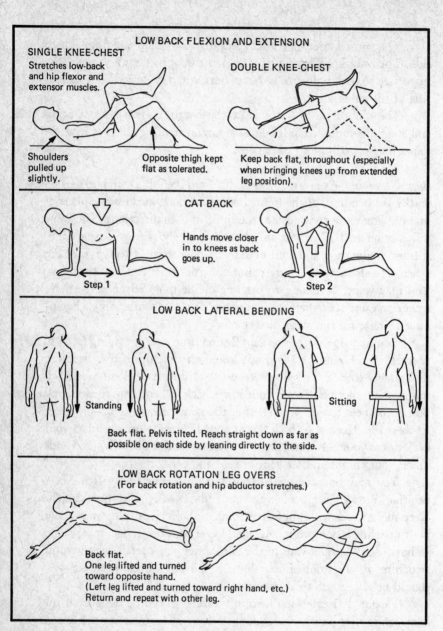

FIGURE 11. Flexibility Exercises for the Back.

cat. (See Figure 11.) Don't use sudden snapping movements. Doing this exercise is a good way to get the feel of lumbar flexion and extension. The same motions can be done from a side-lying position or seated on a stool, once you are used to the feel of them.

The most popular back flexion and extension exercise is the standing toe touch. Begin with the hands overhead, arch the back, and then bend forward and try to touch your toes. Keep your knees straight or nearly straight. If you have down-the-leg sciatic pain, you should not try to keep your knees straight while doing this. This exercise should be done in a smooth, controlled fashion. Avoid sudden bursts of effort and bobbing, ballistic repetitions. Standing toe touches are good for those who have conditioned themselves. They are not beginning exercises for back pain sufferers. Begin with lying, kneeling, and seated exercises before proceeding to standing toe touches.

You may do lateral bending exercises for the lower back from a standing position. (See Figure 11.) Alternately slide one hand down the side of your thigh as far toward the knee as you can. Don't twist or bend forward. Do this in a slow, easy, relaxed fashion. The same stretch may be duplicated from the sitting position in a chair or stool. It is harder to gain this motion lying down because the weight of the arm assists you with the stretch. Another form of lateral motion—the side glide—is described in the section on posture exercises.

You can practice rotation of your lower back by doing legovers from the supine position. (See Figure 11.) Lie with your legs straight out and arms to the side at right angles to your body. Lift one leg and bring it across the other and up as far toward the opposite arm as you can. Avoid sudden jerks. Alternate the effort from one side to the other. This puts a twisting stress on your lower back, so you should do it very cautiously. Don't do twisting exercises if you are having sciatic pain. If done in a controlled, cautious fashion, these exercises may help to strengthen the structures that are vulnerable to twisting injury and thereby prevent more serious injury when you twist your back under less controlled circumstances.

Another bending and rotating exercise is a forward-bending toe touch with one foot upon a stool. Slide your hand down the front of the straight leg while keeping the other foot up on the stool with the knee bent. Keep both feet pointed straight ahead. This places a controlled, mild, twisting stress on the lower back. It sometimes can be used as a help, along with side gliding, to correct a list.

A variation on rotation exercise is sometimes called self-traction or self-manipulation. It duplicates the forces placed upon the lower back by a common method used to manipulate or adjust the back. These forces are directed at the facet joints of the lower back. Lie on your side with the most painful side up. Place one or two pillows under your hip and flank. Bring your top leg forward, and draw your knee toward your chest. Allow the weight of your leg and foot to fall in front of your body so that you feel a forward-twisting motion of your pelvis. Next, bring your upper arm behind your back and allow your shoulder to fall backward so that the weight of your arm is behind your body. This can be done for sudden catches as described in the chapter on first aid. It also can be done to maintain the motion in these joints.

Hip and Knee Motion Exercises. Tight muscles along the side of the hip (abductors) can be stretched by legovers. For those who do legovers well and have worked up to more vigorous exercise, the iliotibial band stretch can be incorporated into the stretching program. Stand with your side to a wall at arm's length. Support your weight against the wall with your outstretched arm and hand. Slowly bend your elbow, keeping your knees straight and feet together. Allow your body to lean in, side toward the wall, so that you feel the stretch in the muscles along the side of your thigh and hip closer to the wall.

You can stretch the hip adductors (the inside thigh muscles) gently by gradually spreading your legs in the supine position. Active assisted or passive adductor stretching may be more effective. For the well conditioned, the standing adductor stretch may be done by placing the inside of the foot on an elevated surface, such as a chair, table, or exercise bar, and bending the other knee. This takes considerable balance and strength to be safe, and it is certainly not a beginning exercise.

The quadriceps muscles of the front of the thigh are major supporters of the knee. They cross the front of the hip and the knee, so they act to bend the hip and straighten the knee. To stretch the whole muscle group, you have to hold the hips straight and bend the knee. You can do this if you lie on your stomach and pull your foot back toward your buttock. (See Figure 12.) If these muscles are tight, you will be able to see how that tightness contributes to back pain, because as you try to stretch them, your back will want to pull into lordosis. Avoid lordosis when doing this exercise by putting a small pillow under your abdomen. Some people find it easier to stretch the quadriceps muscles while standing. Hold on to something steady with the opposite hand, and use your stomach muscles and a pelvic tilt to avoid lordosis. Then reach back and hold your foot with your hand on the same side, and pull that foot up toward your buttock. You should feel it stretch the front of your hip and knee.

Tight hip flexor muscles frequently accompany tight ligaments in the front of the hip. The quadriceps stretching exercises and the back extension exercises are both needed to relieve tightness across the front of the hip.

The most difficult stiffness problem for many people with low back pain is that of stiff hamstrings. (See Figure 12.) The hamstring muscles cross the back of the hip and the back of the knee and are stretched by bending your hip with your knees straight. Unfortunately, the sciatic nerve takes the same course. It is, therefore, difficult to stretch tight hamstring muscles effectively if your sciatic nerve roots are scarred or sensitive.

Any exercise that results in hip flexion with a straight knee puts stretch on your hamstrings. Lifting your leg with your knees straight requires considerable muscular effort and is better for strengthening than for stretching. If you have someone to hold the weight of your leg while you do this, it is a safer and more effective stretching exercise.

Toe touching with the knees straight is a good hamstring stretch for those who can tolerate it. It should not be done by beginners or those with sciatic pain.

The safest and most controlled means of hamstring stretching is done while sitting in a chair. Keep one leg straight ahead with the knee bent and the foot flat on the floor. Straighten your other leg at the knee,

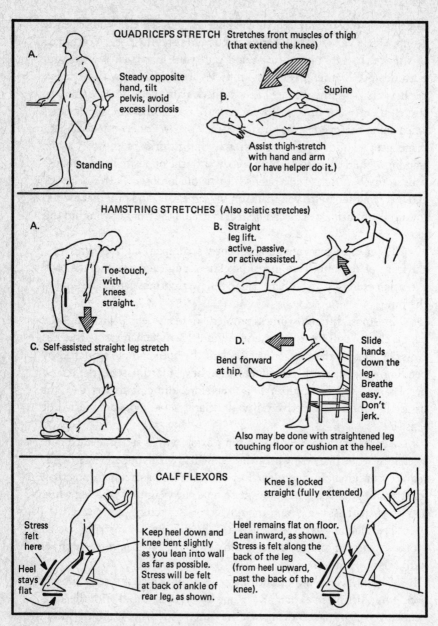

FIGURE 12. Flexibility Exercises for the Legs.

and point the toe of that leg straight ahead. Now lean forward and run both hands down the straight leg. Allow your head to bend toward that knee. This method is safer and gentler because it does not pose a problem with maintaining balance and does not require simultaneous stress to both legs.

You may do a more advanced hamstring stretching exercise from a standing position. Support your weight on one foot with the knees straight. Lift the other leg with the knee bent, and rest the foot on a chair or car bumper. It is best if you have a place to steady one or both hands. Now force the elevated knee straight while you bend forward.

Never do hamstring stretching exercises ballistically. Slow, steady stretches are more effective and much safer. Be especially cautious if you have sciatic pain.

Calf and Ankle Stretching. The calf muscles begin above the knee, join additional muscles that begin below the knee, and then extend as the heel cord (Achilles tendon) across the back of the ankle. The muscles that begin above the knee must be stretched separately from those that begin below the knee. (See Figure 12.)

Stand facing a wall at arm's-length. Support your weight on both hands against the wall. Lift your weight from one leg. Lean into the wall, and keep the heel of the weight-bearing leg on the floor. First keep your knee bent. The pull on the back of the ankle and muscles of the lower calf is from stretch of the muscles that begin below your knee. Now straighten your knee, keeping your heel down. Feel the stretch across the back of the knee as the muscles that begin above the knee are stretched.

If you do calf and ankle stretching barefooted, you also stretch the muscles that cross your foot. If you have pain in those muscles, however, you should stretch them first from a sitting position before applying vigorous stretch to them while standing.

Exercises for General Fitness

Some people seem to be able to work and live under great stress without showing the effects of tension. Some people seem to endure injuries and illnesses that must be very painful without letting pain interfere with their function and enjoyment of life. In some cases, these people are just born with high tolerance to stress and pain. Others seem to develop these abilities.

One of the characteristics of a large percentage of these people is exceptional physical fitness. Witness the pain and discomfort endured by soldiers in battle, football players, boxers, and marathon runners. They may be able to withstand injury at the moment and go on because they are psyched up or their adrenalin is up, but they also seem to suffer less afterward than unfit people with similar injuries. Studies of workers on fitness programs compared to workers who are not so fit show that those who are fit miss far less work from comparable injuries. One such study showed that back injuries were 10 times more frequent among unfit workers than fit workers.

Not only do those that are exceptionally well fit seem to be able to withstand physical injury better, but they also tolerate stress and frustration better, have less trouble with depression, and require less sleep.

All of the reasons for these advantages of fitness are not known. One explanation is that the physical stress of regular exercise produces brain hormones that act to decrease feelings of pain. The psychological benefits of feeling strong and capable of controlling one's body also must play some part.

It has been only in the relatively recent history of humanity that most of us, most of the time, are safe from attack. People's need to defend themselves was well served by body reflexes and reactions that prepared us for fight or flight. These same physical mechanisms are still in our bodies, however, and they still exert their effects when we are stressed. Now, however, the stresses are different, and the solutions, when there are some, don't come from physical fight or flight. If we don't have some physical outlet to allow our body mechanisms to work the way they were made to, we don't have good health.

The sort of fitness that helps with stress and pain tolerance and decreases depression is gained by the same sort of exercise that leads to cardiorespiratory (heart and lung) fitness. These exercises improve lung function, decrease high blood pressure, and decrease the risk of death from heart attack.

Exercises to gain these advantages require at least 30 minutes every other day. They should be painless though slightly stressful. The idea is to work up to and sustain an exercise program that will allow continuous, mildly stressful exercise for 30 minutes or more at a time. This is a lifetime commitment, so you would be foolish to rush into an exercise program too fast and make it unpleasant or risk injury.

The chosen exercise must be something easily controlled and rhythmic. It should be easily accessible on a year-round, regular basis. The exercise should be easily measurable so that the amount of stress may be increased gradually. It must be something that can be continued for the entire exercise session without rest or the need for sudden bursts of extra effort.

The fitness activities that qualify are jogging, swimming, bicycling, aerobic dancing, rowing, and cross-country skiing. Variations of each of these activities may be most suitable to individuals, but whatever exercise is chosen must conform to the above criteria. You may combine the activities, doing one on one day and another the next, though you need a higher degree of fitness to be able to gain a comparable benefit from combinations of exercises than from one.

Cycling, Rowing, Skiing, and Running at Home. Bicycling, rowing, and cross-country skiing require more apparatus and preparation and place greater demands on time and location than the other activities. These problems can be overcome somewhat, for those who wish to pursue it, by buying home, indoor, stationary exercise equipment that simulates the stress of the activity. For those who need or wish to exercise indoors, these are good alternatives. For those who tolerate exercise best if weight bearing is not required, the stationary bicycle may be the best choice.

You may buy treadmills for home use so you can run indoors. A similar device is available that allows you to duplicate the movements of cross-country skiing. The expense, space requirement, and maintenance of large and complex equipment are the major drawbacks.

Small, trampoline-like jogging platforms are simple devices for running, jumping, or doing dance exercises at home. The problem with the elastic jogging platforms is that the elastic produces a lot of movement, which may give you the feeling that you are doing more exercise than you really are. You must monitor your breathing or pulse rates to make sure you are expending sufficient effort to help you. You must also take care to avoid injury from losing your balance while exercising on an elastic platform.

Swimming. Swimming may be used for muscle strengthening, for general fitness, or for both. Strengthening requires bursts of near maximum effort, which, if done properly, could not be sustained for long enough to serve as a fitness exercise. Fitness, conversely, requires prolonged, sustained effort. The strokes may be the same, but the intensity and duration of effort are different.

Swimming is excellent fitness activity if the effort is continuous. You cannot stop for breaks at the end of the pool or interrupt the exercise with any sort of rest. Though it may be possible to sustain the effort for only a few minutes at first, the goal to maintain fitness is more than 30 minutes of continuous, moderately stressful effort at each workout.

The neck stress of taking breaths from prolonged effort at free-style swimming can be avoided by using a snorkel and goggles so that the head is kept beneath the water.

The breast stroke requires a lot of neck extension, lumbar lordosis, and rapid shifts in low back position. Side arm (elementary) back stroke, while not a competitive swim stroke, places least stress on the low back. It is the best stroke for those with neck or back pain who are working into swimming as a fitness activity.

The biggest problems with swimming as a fitness activity are its seasonal nature and finding regular access to a pool where uninterrupted distance swimming is possible. Remember, to gain full benefits from a fitness program, you must exercise at least every other day. Consequently, most people who include distance swimming in their fitness program use it as a supplemental exercise and depend upon one of the more easily accessible activities for their regular fitness workouts.

To be satisfactory for fitness exercise, swimming pools require a long enough straightaway, with depth to allow for swimming laps back and forth without stopping. To be satisfactory for water flexibility and strengthening exercise, swimming pools need to have a standing surface where water is at chest level and armholds are available on the sides.

Aerobic Dancing and Calisthenics. In 1969 Dr. Kenneth Cooper's book, *Aerobics,* described a series of exercises designed to be done for continuous, relatively long periods without becoming breathless. Jacki Sorensen adapted aerobic exercises to music and coined the term *aerobic dance.* Though there is a specific program designed by Sorensen's Aerobic Dance, Inc., the term aerobic dance is generally used to refer to any series of sustained, choreographed movements done for the purpose of providing general fitness.

Dancing and calisthenic forms of exercises certainly have some great advantages. Most communities have professionals who will lead groups through these types of fitness programs at reasonable cost. The use of music or rhythmic chanting makes the exercise more pleasant for some. The social aspects of group activity and the encouragement you get from fellow exercisers may be big pluses.

Most programs can be adapted easily to home use, so you don't need to be with the group on days when you would rather exercise at home alone.

You must take some precautions if you choose one of the variations of aerobic dancing or calisthenics to be your fitness activity. Most leaders of these groups are exceptionally fit and physically capable people who have and can generate a lot of enthusiasm for exercising. It is very easy for them to lead their followers to push beyond the level for which they are ready. Most programs require that the instructors be fit individuals who know how to monitor stress and perform cardio-pulmonary resuscitation. It would be ideal if they were qualified to identify specific exercise problems, advise about precautions, and set appropriate limits for each individual, but such ideals are not often available. Observe a session or two before you contract with a supervised exercise group. Try to find an instructor who will be patient with your limitations and a group which has age, fitness levels, and goals similar to your own. You must remind yourself that what you are seeking is lifetime fitness and that, though you want to progress steadily, pushing too fast is not worth the risk of injury or discouragement.

Another problem with aerobic dancing is that the action may be noncontinuous. Aerobic means that you do not get out of breath during the activities. In fact, if you are exercising properly, your breathing effort increases so that you are breathing faster and deeper than you normally would. Your breathing does not increase to the point where you feel you have no reserve and must slow way down or stop. You want to reach a plateau where you are breathing more deeply and faster than normal, but where, with an effort, you can continue throughout without slowing down the exercise. If the exercises are done with an effort so that you become breathless during one exercise and then stop and catch your breath before going to the next, you are not gaining the sort of general fitness benefit discussed here. Aerobic dancing and calisthenics can be tailored easily to provide smooth and rapid transition from one activity to the next without sudden bursts and rests. That is the way this exercise should be done for the results you are seeking.

Aerobic dance exercises may tend to be ballistic. The rhythm, the music, and the enthusiasm to stay with the group may induce you to make jerking efforts to complete each movement. This jerking is more likely to produce muscle injury. You should be careful to keep your breathing relaxed without breath-holding strains and to keep the muscular effort smooth.

If you stay away from these pitfalls and make sure that none of them results in depriving you of the full benefit of a fitness program or leads you to injury, then the music, the companionship, the variety of movements, and the adaptability of this form of fitness program may make it the most desirable.

Walking, Jogging, and Running. By far, the most popular general fitness activity is some variation of jogging. Whether it is walking, jogging, or speed running depends on the level of fitness and experience of the participant.

For those unaccustomed to regular exercise lasting 30 minutes or more without a break, the thought of running for that long may sound very unappealing. But it does not have to be unpleasant.

The reason why running is selected more than any other form of fitness exercise is because of its simplicity. Running requires very little equipment and very little need to compromise for location or weather. The exercise can be done almost any time it can be fitted into the day, so it requires little planning or preparation.

Not only is jogging the fitness activity selected by the most people, but it is also the activity that most people stick with. More people who have shown that they accept fitness as a lifetime commitment, by continuous adherence to an exercise program for a year or more, do it by jogging than by any other activity.

Many people know that they need to commit to a fitness program, but, because they are unfamiliar with it, they are reluctant and a little afraid. They may try to satisfy themselves that they have made an effort by buying some equipment or outfits or enrolling in a course or group. Those things are all right, but they don't give you what you need. You need commitment and dedication to persist through the fears and some unpleasant aspects of exercising. That is the hard but simple concept. Those that accept it frequently choose the simplest activity, which is jogging.

Some people have back conditions that make prolonged weight-bearing exercise undesirable. An alternative exercise may have to be selected in some cases, but many people who believed they would never be able to run for exercise because of a back condition have been surprised at their success. Many who have begun with an alternative exercise have switched to running as they developed confidence.

Many people believe from personal experience, and many people will tell you, that running is very unpleasant. There are times when you misjudge and push too hard at anything, and those times are unpleasant, but running does not have to be unpleasant.

Becoming breathless is unpleasant. Feeling nauseous is unpleasant. Having stomach cramps is unpleasant. These are symptoms of pushing beyond the level of fitness. They do not have to be and should not be common features of a program of running for fitness.

The mistake made by almost everyone who finds running unpleasant, who gets hurt or sick from running, or who gets discouraged with it is that too much is done too soon. That is a foolish, pointless error that makes your fitness project unpleasant and results in lack of progress.

You want always to be making very gradual progress. You want to think in terms of months rather than days. If you are doing very slightly better than you were last month, that is just right. If you have not been on a fitness program before, whether you know it or not, you have been getting very gradually worse in your cardiorespiratory ability each month for all of your adult life. If you have reversed the direction of those changes, you have done a great thing. Your job is to keep the direction of your fitness toward improvement, never to let it turn around the other way again. The rapidity of the progress is not important. If you get discouraged or hurt and quit, your state of fitness will turn direction and start getting worse. So don't take chances—keep the progress very slow, keep it pleasant, keep it safe, but keep it going.

Most people who are not already running for exercise should begin a jogging fitness program by walking. Walk a distance that is very mildly stressful for you, more than you would walk at one time during the ordinary day but a distance that you are quite sure you can walk without having pain and stiffness afterward. Do gentle flexibility exercises right before and more vigorous ones afterward. Note the distance and the time it took you. Walk at a comfortable pace. Don't try to hurry, but remember that these exercise periods are to be uninterrupted, so don't stop to rest or talk. If you wish, have someone walk with you. Even after you work up to running, you will want to have enough breathing reserve to be able to talk while you run.

For most people, fitness sessions every other day work best. If you have the time and the desire, you can exercise every day and perhaps progress a little faster. Both the good and the bad effects of fitness exercise add up, though, so you must be more careful not to hurt yourself if you exercise every day. Even on an every-other-day schedule, you must remember that you can do far more once than you can do regularly. You should not try to increase your level of exercise until you have demonstrated for at least a week that you can maintain your present level without pain and unpleasantness.

So, for at least the first week, continue to take the same walk you took the first day. If, after that time, you are suffering no ill effects from the walking, increase the distance a little. Never make sudden, dramatic increases. At any level of fitness, it is not advisable to increase your exercise total for the week by more than 10 percent.

This means that if you walk 1.0 mile at each session the first week, you should increase to only about 1.1 mile at each session the second week. Another way of increasing effort that enables you to add variety to the sessions is to add the extra effort to just one or two sessions. For example, if you walked 1.0 mile for each of the first four sessions, you could walk the next four at 1.0, 1.2, 1.0, and 1.2, thus only increasing by 10 percent over the week but adding an occasional longer effort. Keep some balance, though—don't ever try to do the whole week's effort in one day.

Once you have progressed to the point where you can walk three miles at each session without unpleasantness and painful after-effects, you are ready to begin to increase your speed. Take a watch for a few days and check the time it takes you to walk three miles at the comfortable pace you have been using. If you are walking over the same course at the same effort, you will find that the times are fairly constant.

Once you have found the predictable, average time that three miles takes you, begin to try to beat that time. Fifteen to 30 seconds faster is plenty of improvement. Don't try to cut more time off at each session.

Keep lowering the time each week. If you get sore muscles, ease off, just try to stay even for a while, and then start up again with the progress. Be sure to stretch any sore muscles carefully each session. If one spot is consistently troublesome, put ice wrapped in towels on it for 20 to 30 minutes after each exercise.

Once you have gotten the time that it takes for you to cover the three miles so low that you feel you cannot walk any faster, you are ready to begin running. The difference between running and walking is that, with running, for an instant neither foot is in contact with the ground, whereas walkers always have some contact. Running, of course, allows you to get there faster, though some people walk faster than others can run. In fact, you can learn to walk very rapidly, but at a certain point picking up speed by running is less effort than trying to walk faster. Your body will tell you when you have reached that point, and that is when you should begin to run a portion of the distance.

Precautions about Fitness Exercise. If you proceed with a very gradual increasing fitness schedule such as the one suggested here, the precautions are pretty well built into the program. Of course, people with heart disease or other serious illness that might limit exercise tolerance should obtain their doctors' blessings before beginning any fitness program.

Two commonly used methods monitor the level of stress that an exercise is producing. Breathing should be definitely deeper and more rapid than normal but not so much so that conversation cannot be maintained. If you are breathing so hard that you cannot talk comfortably, you need to slow down.

The other method requires taking the pulse. This can be done in the usual way at the wrist. While exercising, counting the carotid pulse in the front of the neck may be easier. Subtract your age from 220, and then take 75 percent of that to obtain the target pulse. For example, if you are age 40, 220 minus 40 equals 180. Then, 180 times 0.75 equals 135. This is the rate at which maximum safe fitness is being obtained. If the rate is above that, you are going too fast; if it is more than 15 beats below the target, you could afford to pick it up a little bit.

These stress monitors are used most often by those who are well along with a fitness program and are trying to keep their progress going as fast as they safely can. When you are first starting, many physical and psychological factors are not accounted for by these monitoring methods. The beginner does best to stay within the limits imposed by these methods but not to push hard to maintain a target pulse right at first. If the pulse gets too fast, you must slow down, but if the pulse is lower than the target pulse, don't worry about it until you have accommodated yourself to the exercise. Just keep trying, keep things going in the right direction without injury, and don't worry, at first, about the speed of progress.

Summary

These discussions of various forms of exercise may seem overwhelming. No one who has many other things to do could do all these exercises, you may think. There is some truth in that, but consider several things that may relieve your anxieties about exercise.

Very few people do all of these exercises all the time. Learning them and working into the usefulness of them takes more time and effort than regular maintenance. As you do the exercises, you will find what you need to work on the most and can concentrate your effort on what is most effective.

People successfully maintain exercise programs without going through all of every routine every day. Flexibility exercises take a few minutes in the morning and in the evening and a few seconds periodically throughout the day. The general fitness sessions require about an hour every other day and can be done morning, noon, or night, as convenient. Follow the general fitness exercise with flexibility exercises. The strengthening exercise can be done on the days that general fitness is not done. The relaxation exercises take some extra time to learn at first, but, once learned, they can be worked into the day whenever they seem to be needed. Few people on a maintenance program spend more than an hour a day doing exercises.

Most of all, you will find, once you are exercising, that you have more time for the rest of your life even if you are investing an hour a day in exercise. If you feel better, can concentrate better on your other tasks, spend less time in hospitals and doctors' offices, spend less time unable to do what you want because you are down, and require less sleep, you will find that when you used to think you didn't have time for exercise, you were losing your chance for more time to be happy and productive.

12
DISABILITY: THE SOCIAL ASPECTS OF BACK PAIN

The interface between legal and work-related problems and the symptom of back pain is terribly complex. It is the most elusive and the single most expensive medical problem confronted by those who make and interpret laws and by those who guide the course of industry.

Part of the problem lurks in the characterization of back pain as a symptom. Clearly demonstrated back problems, such as fractures of the spine, are more predictable, and the needed legal and economic adjustments are easier to calculate. Most people with back pain, however, cannot be given such a precise anatomic diagnosis. The underlying and contributory causes, the role of injury, the effects of treatment, the effects of psychological and social adjustments, and the anatomical and functional outcomes are all uncertain.

The social and economic problems of back pain vary among different regions and countries. Each attempt to analyze the problems is frought with sampling error. Every observer brings the bias of personal experience to the analysis. Each individual included in the analysis has multiple factors of psychological and physical makeup, which influence the way back pain is presented. There are variations in the forces and mechanisms of every injury. The available medical and scientific knowledge is fragmentary, so big gaps are present between what is known about the back and the effects of specific stresses.

There is an abundance of information available, but that doesn't always constitute knowledge. In fact, there is so much conflicting information that one can refer to published statistics to support almost any opinion on any side of any issue surrounding the back pain problem.

Back pain may affect the social and economic lives of people because of decisions about disability or retirement insurance, personal injury suits, or workers' compensation claims. There are other ways, but these are the most common and will be the subjects of this chapter. To understand any of those issues, you must understand the term *disability*.

Most people have a vague notion that disability means an inability to do something, perhaps because of some physical handicap. If pressed to give a precise definition, most would feel a lot of uncertainty about the exact meaning. They should not feel badly; experts don't use the term precisely either. Virtually every time a lawyer and an orthopedic surgeon talk to each other about it, they must stop and define exactly what the other means.

One very proper meaning of the term is the lay person's sense of some handicap or inability to perform some function that is not well defined. That use serves well in everyday conversation. It is very hard, however, to administrate social justice when the issue is so vague. Attempts to treat all parties fairly require that the meaning be clarified in terms that can be quantified—that numbers be assigned to provide information about the amount of disability.

One measure of disability is the percentage of physical impairment. A percentage figure that reflects the degree to which the body is handicapped is assigned. Such percentages can be well defined and agreement can be reached among various parties with relative ease when the diagnosis is precise—an amputation, for example. When the diagnosis is imprecise, as is usually the case with back pain, the percentages are more arbitrary.

Another way to assign numbers to the question of an individual's disability is to consider the monetary cost, usually in terms of lost wages. Such a figure may be very different from the impairment rating because it takes into account such factors as the education, training, and experience of the individual and how some psychological and other social factors may relate to the problem. For example, the loss of a little finger would disable a concert pianist severely, whereas it would result in little or no problem for a lawyer. The physical impairments are the same, but the disabilities judged by other parameters differ greatly.

Disabilities may change with time, treatment, and rehabilitation. Some physical impairments can be reasonably expected to interfere permanently with function or to pose a constant threat of doing so, while others may be more reasonably expected to be temporary and to resolve with time and treatment. Some physical impairments can be reasonably expected to limit wage-earning capacities permanently, whereas others may not. Administration of justice requires a prediction of whether the problem will be temporary or permanent.

Some disabilities may be sufficiently severe to be considered total, either temporary or permanent. This may seem to be a simple extension of the question of the percentage of impairment, but the difference between total disability and partial disability may have special implications under some circumstances. It may depend upon whether the judgment is based on the ability to do any kind of work, any work that would produce substantial gain, any work the individual could be trained to do, or the specific job that the individual had been doing before.

Not all of these factors are important in every circumstance, but generally the distinctions that must be made are whether temporary or permanent, whether total or partial, the percentage of physical impairment, and the percentage of functional disability. The next question to be asked is, "Who decides?"

No one knows more than you how much pain you have. No one knows as well as you what you can do and what you cannot do. Why not, then, allow people to judge for themselves how disabled they are? That would work if everyone were perfectly honest, could judge their problems relative to those of others, and could predict the future for themselves. Such an ideal doesn't exist, however, and those who tried to judge themselves honestly would be left without just compensation from a system impoverished by the dishonest. Many people fear a worse future than they should. Fear to try to function normally is a great hindrance to recovery of normal function, so many people would do a great injustice to themselves by accepting the role of being disabled when they still had potential for normal function.

Most doctors are only willing to provide opinions about the medical aspects of disability, about physical impairment. Most medical specialists will only give opinions about the aspects of impairment that fall within their specialty, so complex medical problems may require opinions from more than one doctor just to arrive at an impairment rating. Translation of that to a disability rating is left to administrators or legal tribunals. Some doctors who consider themselves experts at making disability judgments will consider the individual's education, training, experience, psychological makeup, and social status, along with the physical impairment, and render an opinion about disability. Most doctors think their own training, experience, and psychological makeups do not allow them to breach the gap between impairment and disability. Often, the administrators and legal tribunals do not consider medical doctors qualified to make disability judgments and will ask them to limit their opinions to physical impairment.

Doctors usually are asked to determine what the permanent effects of an injury or an illness are likely to be. When such a prediction can be made will vary depending upon circumstances. With many back problems, there always will be some uncertainty about the future, so reasons can be found to delay the judgment about permanent impairment for a long time. There are, however, often very good reasons, including preservation of the physical health of the individual, to hasten rehabilitation. That may require that the impairment judgment be made as soon as practical.

In the United States, most such judgments are made about nine months after back injuries. Some of that delay is because of uncertainty about the medical outcome, but much of it is administrative. The legal process, where the concern is economic and social consequence, moves at a slower pace than the medical process, sometimes to the disadvantage of the patient.

Everyone wants this process to be as fair as possible. To ensure that, the process may involve many people. The opposing sides are allowed to present their points of view as adversaries. All of this takes time. Sometimes the most important thing at the center of all this concern— the health of the individual—may suffer from the delays caused by everyone's anxiety that everything be done exactly right.

The percentage of impairment that a physician will assign to a given problem depends upon his or her findings from a history and physical examination. X rays and other tests also may be considered.

Many physicians adhere to the principle that their impairment ratings are based only upon objective findings. Objective findings are under the control of the examiner and independent of the history or cooperation of the examinee. An abnormal reflex is objective, whereas a complaint of pain limiting an effort to bend is subjective. Many findings, such as loss of sensation or limited tolerance to movement, may have both subjective and objective elements, so that an experienced examiner may consider some findings as objective even though there is an element of control by the examinee.

Many examiners will rate a physical impairment as zero if there are no objective findings. Some examiners will assign some impairment rating even if there are no objective findings if they believe the subjective findings warrant it. An impairment rating is a statement of what the physician has found that indicates there will be a permanent problem. It is not a statement of whether the physician believes the examinee is telling the truth about his or her pain. Many patients become frustrated with their physicians because they do not understand that.

In spite of all of these variables, there is reasonable conformity in the judgments that most medical doctors make about back conditions. Percentages usually are assigned in terms of impairment to the whole body. Most back conditions with some objective manifestation of permanence are assigned impairment ratings within the range of 5 to 25 percent of the body. Studies from both the United States and Canada show similar practices. The lower numbers in that range are assigned when the condition is perceived to have produced less permanent loss of function, to be likely to produce less permanent problems with pain, and to have better long-range outcome. Higher numbers reflect the examiner's opinion that more permanent pain and loss of function are likely.

It is common for two or more examiners to render different percentages of physical impairment. It is then an administrative or judicial function to decide which impairment rating to accept or to make a compromise, and then to translate the physical impairment rating into a disability rating.

The impairment or disability percentage may be the basis of a settlement of damages awarded by a workers' compensation commission; it may serve as a guideline for government agencies in determination of employability; it may serve for insurance adjusters and injured parties to reach a settlement; it may be a means of supplying a brief and quantitative opinion to a judge or jury; and it may serve as a basis for distinguishing the degree of preexisting difficulty if a future incident occurs.

Sometimes such a percentage figure may be meaningless and unnecessary. It may even be detrimental. Some individuals may take it as a permanent sentence of limitation on their activities and allow it to interfere with complete rehabilitation. The stamp of such a number may close avenues of opportunity. Such harmful confusion of the common, everyday meaning of the term *disability* with the legal meaning can be avoided if assignments of percentage are not made unnecessarily and if the individual has a clear understanding of the different meanings.

Disability judgments are often needed to determine eligibility for private disability insurance, eligibility for early retirement with pension benefits, or eligibility for government-sponsored pensions such as the American Social Security Administration disability benefits program. Veterans' benefit programs, fitness for military service, and physical qualifications for certain jobs are among other needs for such judgments. The circumstances of such needs are different from when the question involves compensation for personal injury.

Private Disability Insurance and Pension Plans

Many people purchase insurance policies that guarantee them certain benefits if they are unable to continue to work because of illness or injury. Such policies are part of some employee benefit packages. There are many variations in the benefits and exclusions of such policies. Many people do not have a clear idea of the terms of their policies. Even when the wording of the policy seems clear, the interpretation may be fuzzy when an issue arises. Back pain is often such a fuzzy issue.

If the policy makes a distinction between benefits provided for injury and those provided for illness, the definition of how those terms apply to a back condition may become important. Some back problems—fractures, for example—are clearly related to a single injury and have nothing to do with illness. Other back conditions, such as certain kinds of arthritis, are clearly illnesses and not injuries. A very large proportion of back problems falls somewhere in between.

If an automobile tire blows out when it rolls over a stone, is the contact with the stone an injury that caused the blowout? Maybe. It depends on the state of the tire, the size of the stone, many other conditions, and the definition of the terms. This example is used to simplify the concept. When applied to the events that may have led to back pain, the judgment is obscured even more by variations in details.

The judgment of whether the back condition is an injury or an illness is based upon the information provided by the individual, by any appropriate witnesses, by the medical records, and by medical opinion. The decision is made by an insurance company administrator or, if necessary, by a court.

Most policies clearly define when benefits begin and for how long they continue. Those dates, however, often are tied to the date on which the individual became unable to work or became able to return to work. Those dates are often sources of controversy. Medical opinion most often provides the basis for decisions of this type, but if there is more than one medical opinion, there may be conflict.

Most policies have a waiting period before benefits begin. Waiting periods may discourage short absences from work. Sometimes, however, they may encourage people to remain out for longer than they should in order to qualify for benefits.

Some policies specify that benefits are to be provided only for total inability to do any kind of work. Others cover partial disabilities or inability to do specific kinds of work. Some list specific partial disabilities. Usually, if specific types are listed, they can be very clearly defined by objective medical criteria, such as amputations and blindness, and do not include the hard-to-define problems like back pain.

Back conditions usually are considered a partial disability. Whether or not the partial disability from a back condition renders an individual unable to work at the specific job that was held may be the point of controversy for some policies. Whether such a condition renders the individual unable to do some work for which he or she would be eligible by education and experience may be another controversial point. The differences depend upon the terms of the policy and how those terms are interpreted by the insurance carrier or, if contested, by the courts.

Controversy occurs when the person with back pain thinks that the pain is too severe to permit work, the doctor says there isn't enough medical evidence to judge the patient unable to work, and the insurance company says that if the doctor says some work is permissible, then benefits are not allowed. If no compromise is made between these conflicting stances, and the individual sues for the benefits of the policy, the matter must be submitted to the courts.

Questions of eligibility for pension benefits for employees who retire early because of a medical disability present a similar set of circumstances. The most common controversies that arise over pension benefits involve employees who are within a few years of normal retirement age. Their pension contract has some provision for benefits to begin if retirement is early because of illness or injury. Often, the job is a physically difficult one. Under those circumstances, the employer or the immediate supervisor may be encouraging the applicant to retire early. The applicant has back pain, but medical examinations often show findings consistent with aging rather than a specific disease or effect of injury. This may not, therefore, meet the requirements of the pension contract.

The danger to applicants for disability benefits is that they may take steps that endanger their physical and economic health and never receive any benefits. In order to obtain benefits they believe they deserve, some people are led to exaggerate their problems. They may miss more work than would have been necessary and thereby alienate themselves from their employers. They may request more medical examination and treatment and state their symptoms in a more dramatic manner than they otherwise would have done. Their medical complaints may have led to more tests and more treatments than they should have had. Those tests and treatments may have made the back problems worse, psychologically if not physically. If the terms of their contracts did not call for benefits for the problem they had, they may have risked their physical and social well-being for nothing.

Social Security Disability

Most governments of industrialized nations provide some forms of pension benefits for retired persons. Citizens may become eligible for such benefits if they become physically unable to work at a preretirement age. In the United States, those benefits are administered by the Social Security Administration.

Applicants for such benefits frequently give back pain as the reason why they are unable to work. In Sweden, 25 percent of new government pension cases are for back pain. In the United States, back pain ranks second only to mental illness as a cause for receiving government disability benefits by those under age 40, and for those over 40 it ranks third behind heart disease and arthritis.

In the past two decades, it has become apparent that the cost of such programs is a significant social problem. In the 15-year span beginning in 1960, the number of people receiving such benefits in the United States increased by eight times. In the 15 years beginning in 1965, the benefits paid through the Social Security Administration for permanent total disability increased from $1.6 billion to $17.2 billion.

The response of governments that have felt overburdened by the costs of these programs has been to try to limit distribution of the benefits. Terms of total disability have been defined more stringently. Enforcement has been more strict. Periodic recertification has been required of those already receiving benefits. Monetary awards have been reduced.

There is considerable variation among different nations regarding who is eligible for such benefits, how much benefits are received, and how continued eligibility is monitored. These are politically explosive issues, so the laws change frequently. Enforcement of the laws varies considerably with local interpretation and in response to political and administrative pressures. Some American states have two and a half times as many people receiving social security disability benefits as others, a figure determined somewhat by local economic factors but also by local administrative practices.

In the United States, eligibility for social security disability benefits requires that the applicant be unable to work for at least one year. There must be documented physical findings that would lead to a reasonable presumption that the applicant would not be able to engage in substantial gainful activity for that period of time.

Enforcement of those criteria have been somewhat uneven, but the spiraling expense of this program has led to more rigid adherence in recent years. Doctors have been asked to spell out in greater detail what objective findings would contribute to inability to work. Applicants have been asked to submit to more thorough and more frequent medical examinations. Administrative decisions have been less lenient.

It has been recognized in the United States and elsewhere that a very large percentage of young (and, therefore, potentially long-duration) recipients of these benefits have been eligible based on disorders such as back pain and mental illness for which evaluation is subjective and determination of work capacity is arbitrary. Those diagnostic groups may be subject to more attention and strict adherence to eligibility requirements by administrators who are under pressure to reduce costs.

In the United States, recertification is required. That means that once benefits are awarded, the recipient must submit to periodic medical examinations to document continuing inability to work. Such a requirement presents the possibilities that benefits may be discontinued because of improvement in the medical condition or because of changes in laws or enforcement policies.

Most people are in favor of such programs. There are many people in desperate need of the benefits. There are two major criticisms. One is that, unless the benefits are carefully restricted to those who really need them, the program becomes inordinately expensive. The other is that such programs provide disincentives to those who otherwise would find some way to do for themselves and in so doing would live happier, healthier lives than they do as disability benefit recipients.

Some people are encouraged to apply for such benefits by friends or family who are attracted by the supplemental income. Some are encouraged by employers who no longer have use for them at the work place. Some see others who seem to be less impaired than they are and yet are receiving benefits.

Many people pursue the idea of receiving such benefits without a good understanding of the erosion of their sense of psychological well-being that occurs if they accept the role of a disability recipient when there is still some potential for them to be gainfully employed. The rewards of being as healthy and self-sufficient as we can be are well worth the struggle. It is a tragic situation when a well-meaning social program discourages an individual from that pursuit.

Disability and Personal Injury

If you think you have been damaged because of someone's negligence, you may file a suit to recover payment for damages from the negligent party. Such a negligent act is called a tort, and the section of the legal and judicial structure that deals with it is called the tort system. Through the tort system, the law seeks to resolve disputes so that injured parties can be compensated for their losses by those responsible for the injury.

The plaintiff, the one seeking payment for damages, must prove four things to recover damages from the defendant. The plaintiff must prove that there was indeed an injury, that as a result of that injury loss occurred, that the injury was the result of the defendant's negligence, and that the plaintiff had not himself or herself contributed to causing the injury. Each of these may be a point of contention to be argued between the plaintiff and the defendant.

Medical testimony addresses the issues of whether or not an injury did indeed occur and what were the losses in terms of physical impairment. The physician may be placed in a difficult circumstance. If the plaintiff has chosen the physician to provide care, the plaintiff expects the physician to be sympathetic. If the plaintiff is engaged in an adversarial relationship with the defendant concerning the medical condition, the plaintiff expects the physician's allegiance. The physician feels a sympathy for and an allegiance with the patient as a patient but not with the patient as a litigant. The physician must, because of his or her personal and professional integrity and because of the mandate of the legal system, be neutral in a situation where all of the other parties take sides. Many patient–plaintiffs do not understand that and resent it, and as a result they seek more and different medical examinations and treatments, sometimes to their detriment.

In the tort system, damages may be awarded for pain and suffering. The impairment rating, which usually reflects the objective observations of physical change in the patient's body, may be relatively less important if a substantial portion of the damages the plaintiff is seeking is for pain and suffering. The physician's description of any specific objective findings that would tend to document that an injury did indeed occur may be more important than a percentage rating.

Back pain is difficult for the physician to evaluate when there are no clear, objective signs. Most experienced physicians are good at sensing how much pain their patients are having. They use that good sense in deciding what diagnostic tests to do and what treatments to order, but they find it difficult to describe or quantify it for legal purposes. Most physicians are very reluctant to say that a patient is lying and not really in pain, though they may sense that at times.

Physicians recognize that patients sometimes may be coached by legal counsel, friends, or family to present certain symptoms or request certain tests or treatments. This is a fact of the adversarial system. It doesn't mean the patient's other complaints aren't valid or that a significant medical condition does not exist, but it makes it more difficult for the physician to render good care.

Many tort actions require testimony from physicians other than the plaintiff's treating physician. The testimony of one or more specialists may be necessary. Testimony may be desirable from physicians who are disinterested. Even though the treating physician may try to be neutral, he or she may not be able to divorce himself or herself completely from his or her allegiance to the patient, or it may be difficult for the physician to take a purely objective look at the final consequences of an injury he or she has been involved with all along.

It is common practice for the plaintiff to submit to an examination by a physician of the defendant's choosing. Some physicians have attitudes and practices of interpretation that are more regularly favorable to plaintiffs and some that are more so for defendants. Most medical specialists consciously try to avoid partiality, but there are honest individual differences that make one doctor different from another in those respects. These differences sometimes become known among defense and plaintiff attorneys. Most often, those differences are small and become important only for balance in an adversarial situation.

One of the problems with the tort system is that the conclusion is often very slow in coming. Many people become concerned enough about the proceedings of such actions that they allow their lives to be altered significantly while this sometimes very protracted course unfolds. The patient–plaintiff may feel a conflict of interest between returning to work, adhering to medical recommendations, enjoying life, and otherwise behaving in a normal fashion on the one hand and the progress of the suit on the other.

Medical testimony will come from the treating physician, who has a good sense of the severity of the problem. Repeated requests for unnecessary examinations or treatments and exaggerations of the problem are not apt to change the treating physician's testimony very much. The testimony of medical examiners asked to give additional opinions is likely to be based upon objective standards. The differences in medical testimony will dilute and balance one another. The risks that some people take and the degree to which they allow their lives to be disrupted by becoming overly involved with the pursuit of payment for tort damages are clearly not worth the tiny influence their actions have on medical testimony.

Workers' compensation laws made major modifications to the tort system. Passage of these laws has been called the most dramatic event in the history of modern civil justice.

During the Industrial Revolution, workers were placed at a disadvantage when they tried to receive just compensation for injuries received at work. The changes in work conditions and the emphasis on productivity had made it more likely that injuries would occur. Attempts at justice through the tort system threatened the efficiency that was necessary to the survival of the new industrialism. This led to some compromises meant to benefit both employers and employees.

Germany had a workers' compensation law in 1884, and Great Britain had one in 1887. By 1908, all western industrialized nations had some form of workers' compensation law. American courts, citing infringement on individual freedoms, were reluctant to accept such laws, but by 1920 the more hazardous occupations were covered in the United States. There have been great variations among the states, but the acceptance of the concept has evolved slowly. By 1950, all American states had provisions for workers' compensation coverage for the majority of workers.

In 1970, the U.S. government passed the Occupational Safety and Health Act. Among other provisions, it established a National Commission on State Workman's (even at that late date, the sexist designation had not disappeared from the lexicon) Compensation Laws, which eventually suggested 19 reforms. If enacted by all the states, they would broaden considerably the scope of problems covered by workers' compensation laws. Approximately 90 percent of American workers are now covered. Of those covered, 65 percent are by private insurance companies, 25 percent by government programs, and the rest by self-insuring industry.

To extend coverage where it was not met adequately by state provisions, the U.S. government passed the Federal Employees' Compensation Act, the Longshoremen's and Harbor Workers' Compensation

Act, the Federal Employees Liability Act (which covers railway workers), and the Federal Coal Mine Health and Safety Act. The last established a particularly significant precedent. It broadens coverage to provide for illness that may arise from exposure to ordinary work conditions. Earlier laws limited coverage to injury from extraordinary events.

Workers' compensation legislation was an economic compromise of the traditional rights of both the injured (the employee) and the party who may be charged with responsibility for the injury (the employer). The compromise was made so that the economic system would survive.

The injured employee sacrifices the right to sue for all losses, most specifically for pain and suffering. The employee gains immediate compensation for all medical expenses and reasonable compensation for lost wages and does not have to prove negligence on the part of the employer. The employee is also freed of the burden of being accused of negligence if a coworker is injured while working.

The employer gains a substantial reduction in legal and administrative expense compared to settling such matters through the tort system. Losses are more predictable in a system that excludes arbitrary awards to be paid for pain, suffering, or punitive damages. The adversary relationship between the employer and the injured employee is diminished, and good employer–employee relationships on matters regarding work safety are encouraged. To gain these benefits, the employer accepts responsibility for all work-related injuries and forfeits the immunity that the tort system would provide should the injured not be able to prove that the injury occurred because of a negligent act on the part of the employer.

The system has worked to a point. For many years, industry was well served by the predictable losses and streamlined handling of compensation cases. The workers, who had been at terrible disadvantage in trying to take an adversarial stance against powerful companies, were provided better medical care and better wage loss benefits than they could have hoped for under the nineteenth-century system.

In recent decades, some substantial problems with the system have occurred. It is an enormously complex system, and everyone who looks at it comes away with a different perception depending upon his or her bias and the view he or she has been provided. Like the fable of the blind men describing an elephant, each individual may have a very good picture of one small part, but it is hard for anyone to conceive of the whole thing accurately. Like the elephant, what everyone has come to realize is that it is a very big problem. Some statistics provide an idea of how big a problem it is.

In the United States in 1970, $3.0 billion were awarded in workers' compensation benefits; in 1976, it was $7.6 billion; in 1980, it was $10.0 billion; and in 1982, it was $14.0 billion. That growth in compensation benefits has occurred in a country whose population and work force are not growing rapidly and whose medical and industrial safety skills are excellent. One-third of those benefits are for medical care and two-thirds are for compensation for lost wages. In 1976, that meant that out of every 100 U.S. payroll dollars, $1.80 went for workers' compensation. By 1982, that figure was $2.55.

There is good reason to discuss workers' compensation in a book about back pain. About 25 percent of all compensable injuries are back injuries, and 33 percent of compensation dollars go for back injuries. The U.S. National Center for Health Statistics reports that back injuries are the number one cause of limitations on work activity of those under age 45 and second only to respiratory infection as a cause of lost work time. Back injury is the most expensive illness in the 30-to-60-year-old age group in industrialized nations.

Studies from Great Britain, Canada, Israel, and Sweden all show that about 50 out of every 1000 workers report work-related back injuries each year. Of those, 18 can be expected to be out of work for more than a month and 4 will be out permanently. British, American, and Swedish studies indicate that about 5.5 percent of the work force was out with back pain in 1970 and 8 percent in 1980.

The cost of workers' compensation benefits, just for back injuries, in the United States was $1.9 billion in 1976, $2.6 billion in 1978, and $5.0 billion in 1981. One insurance industry study estimated that workers' compensation cost of low back pain in the U.S. in 1982 at $10 billion. Figures from Great Britain indicate a cost of about 1 million pounds per day.

Certain specific industries have worse records than others. Each time you use an American 20-cent postage stamp, you can figure that about 1.5 cents goes for workers' compensation benefits for the back injuries of postal employees. These costs are just those that can be related directly to benefits. If one considers all of the related costs of lost productivity and efficiency, the bill for back pain in the United States may be around $50 billion per year.

In terms of work days, there are about 90.0 million lost each year in the United States and 13.2 million in Great Britain because of back injuries. A British employer of manual laborers may figure that for every 100 employees, there will be 70 weeks per year off work because of back pain. American estimates indicate that for each 1000 workers, 1400 work days are lost to back pain each year.

Of those who lose work because of back pain, about half will have a recurrence at some time. Of those who are out of work longer than six months, only 50 percent ever return to work. Only 25 percent of those out over a year ever do so.

These statistics should alarm everyone. They reflect threats to current economic systems as well as to the personal welfare of individuals. They are hard to reconcile with the facts that medical care has gotten progressively better and that work place safety measures have improved steadily.

Some statistics suggest that the system may have some self-destructive features. One study of groups of back-injured workers who were and were not covered by workers' compensation found that the back trouble was stated to have originated from a work-related accident by 90 percent of the insured and by 40 percent of the uninsured. Studies that compare the benefits awarded by various compensation schemes indicate that those systems that provide the most liberal benefits have the highest percentage of back-injured workers. These data can be interpreted in several ways, but, along with the other statistics, they show that there is a major problem that seems to be getting worse.

One should not take any of these statistics and point fingers about who is at fault. The question may be more appropriately stated as, "What's at fault?"

Over the past several decades, there has been a growing tendency among health care professionals to look at health problems holistically. The role of stress and the influences of the physical and emotional environment upon the well-being of individuals have been given more attention. The result has been a trend toward redefinition of the term *injury*. The meaning is no longer confined to a single, well-defined event that produces an effect that can be clearly determined to be the result of that event. All contributory factors are considered. That, of course, includes events, even ordinary ones, that occur at work. The extension of that concept so that such injuries are covered under the workers' compensation laws has been commonplace when considering back-pain-related conditions.

Progress in medical science has led to better recognition and understanding of many conditions. As a result of such progress, work-related causes have been identified in some conditions that were not understood previously.

Medical progress has provided more elaborate diagnostic means and more extensive treatment possibilities. Though the costs are offset somewhat by the positive results they produce by returning people to work, they have made the medical bills for workers' compensation enormous.

The concept of rehabilitation of the whole person is consistent with the holistic viewpoint of the causes of illness. It also has greatly expanded the scope and expense of what health care professionals seek to provide for injured workers. The records of medical care paying for itself by more rapid return of the injured to the work force are best when dealing with well-defined acute injury. They are worst with vaguely defined chronic problems. Humanistic considerations, however, demand that adequate medical care be provided regardless of cost-effectiveness.

There has been a general fuzziness of definition of what is and what is not an injury and what conditions are and are not likely to be related to some event that occurred at work. Until very recent years, the trend among physicians, and among legal and administrative interpreters as well, has been toward permissiveness, extending benefits under the cloak of the workers' compensation laws when doubt exists.

These trends and discoveries have provided some needed benefits where they were well deserved. They also may have been abused. Any way you look at it, they have been very expensive.

Another reason why workers' compensation has become more expensive is that there has been some erosion of the original boundaries. Plaintiffs have become more aggressive and courts more permissive in allowing crossovers into the tort system, so that benefits are sometimes sought in both systems. Third-party responsibilities, product liabilities, and joint responsibilities are all issues that may result in more complex litigation effort. This has resulted in a reduction in one of the original benefits of the workers' compensation laws—brief and inexpensive application.

Workers' compensation plans do provide the means to contest decisions, or at least for the parties to be represented and their viewpoints presented by counsel before a final decision is made. If the impairment is temporary, if it is total, and if it is caused by a clearly defined physical limitation such as an amputation, the calculations are often simple and not as likely to be contested. When the injury is less well defined and results in permanent, partial disability, the judgment is arbitrary, less amenable to agreement, and more likely to be contested. The increasing number of workers' compensation claims for back injuries, many of them contested, has encumbered the system with more legal and administrative processes than the design had intended.

Some of the responsibility for the problems with the American workers' compensation programs has been assigned to the administration of various programs. Federal studies have cited uneven application and inadequacies of state-administered programs.

Some of the cost increase of the American system, however, seems to have stemmed from the expense of centralized programs. Workers' compensation costs for those covered under the Longshoremen's Act have risen at a rate six times that of wages. After benefits under the Federal Employees Compensation Act were increased in 1974, there was an eightfold increase in lost time injuries by 1979. The U.S. General Accounting Office estimated that one-third of federal workers would have more take-home pay if they were receiving workers' compensation benefits while not working than they would if they were working.

The United States provides a good model for the study of various workers' compensation systems, since each state is a little different from the others. Some states have claims judged by commissions, and some have courtroom proceedings very similar to those of the tort system.

Most states provide that injured workers receive a portion of their usual wage when they are temporarily unable to work. In most instances, it is about 66 percent. Some states tie the figure to the average worker's wage in that state. Some apportion benefits based upon the difference between the previous wage and what the worker could make working with the present impairment. Some states set a maximum figure that can be paid.

There are variations in the time schedules of benefit payments. Some programs specify that wage loss compensation benefits begin immediately after the injury occurs. Some require that benefits be started only after the employer agrees that the injury is work-related or a judicial decision declares it so. Many programs have a waiting period so that wage loss compensation is paid only after a specified number of days of work have been missed. Many have a limit on the number of weeks that benefits can be received for a specific injury, while others are open-ended or depend on the injured being under active medical treatment.

Many states specify that, after a reasonable period of time or after sufficient medical evidence is available, a permanent settlement must be reached. Such a settlement, often called a compromise and release agreement, provides the injured with a monetary compensation and releases the employer from further obligation to compensate the injured. Such agreements can be for either the wage continuation benefits or the medical benefits or both. They allow the employer to take the loss and be free of the uncertainties of future obligation and the administrative expense of keeping the case open. They provide the injured with immediate benefits and freedom from the emotional drain and continuing uncertainties of an open claim. The disadvantage of such agreements, of course, is that both parties are betting that the compromise at which they arrive proves to be a just one.

The variations among these different workers' compensation provisions demonstrate that there are many possible schemes of awarding wage loss benefits. The cost of the system and the benefits it provides can be varied by adjusting these variables. It is also possible to adjust costs and services by regulation of the legal and medical contributions to the system.

Some workers' compensation agreements specify that the injured be examined and treated only by specific doctors chosen by the employer. Others pay any medical expense from any health care source chosen by the patient. There are all gradations of control between those two extremes. Many will only reimburse the injured for medical expenses from or authorized by a licensed physician and will not pay for care from nonmedical practitioners. Some programs specify or limit the fees that physicians may charge. Some require a second opinion before prolonged or expensive treatments are undertaken.

The original hope of the workers' compensation scheme was that it would be simple. It was the hope that an injured worker who was not sophisticated about legal and bureaucratic process could be justly compensated. Unfortunately, that has not always been the case. Insurance companies aggressively try to limit their losses. Insurors and employers react emotionally to a system in which they see unfair advantage taken of them at times. The reluctant stances of insurors may make it difficult for the legitimate claimant to receive his or her just benefits. When claimants feel they cannot obtain justice, they may seek counsel from an attorney. Attorneys who work in this system can provide their clients with equal footing through the red tape and uncertainties that may overwhelm the unsophisticated.

Attorneys, of course, charge fees for their knowledge and their time. The fee may be a substantial part of the benefit. The claimant, therefore, must decide if he or she is at sufficient disadvantage in the system to make the attorney's fee worth it. There is no question that the average award to a claimant without an attorney is less than the average award to a claimant with an attorney. Some injured parties, however, would have taken home more benefits without their attorneys. The claimant must decide if the employer and the insurance company are dealing fairly enough so that a satisfactory settlement will be reached without an attorney. If not, a judgment must be made to decide if the attorney's fee and the trouble of a suit will be justified by the difference in the settlement.

Because the system has become so complex, more people feel that they are unable to deal with it and hire lawyers to assist them. That has resulted in higher total benefits. More lawyers in the system make the system more complex and expensive. The advantage is that better justice is brought to the deserving claimant.

One way in which system designs may limit the expense and complexity is to limit the role of lawyers. This is often done by building disincentives to lawyers into the system. Limiting the fees that lawyers may receive for such cases is a method under trial in some states. Since the legal fees are already somewhat limited because of the exclusion of pain and suffering benefits from the workers' compensation system, any further limitation makes many lawyers feel the rewards do not justify their efforts. If many lawyers come to feel that way, it may become difficult for a claimant to obtain legal counsel, which would result in a simpler and less expensive system but would cause injustice for some claimants.

Some workers' compensation systems have sought to include vocational rehabilitation as an integral part of the plan. Benefits may be excluded or withheld until the injured is actively participating in a vocational rehabilitation program. The theory is that an injured worker who has been rehabilitated and returned to some job has been well served and is no longer a financial or administrative burden. If the success rate were high, such a program would satisfy both humane and economic needs. If many of the claimants are not highly motivated to return to the work force and if the economy is not calling for additional workers, however, the success rate of vocational rehabilitation services is not likely to be high.

There is no clear evidence to prove what are the right or wrong approaches to workers' compensation administration. Carefully controlled, unbiased social research is certainly needed. At least in America, the available data suggest that the answers must come somewhere in the middle ground between centralized, liberal benefit programs and abandonment of the concept with return to the tort system. While the traditional judicial process is too slow and expensive to serve as a permanent solution, one hope is that those issues that have been taken through judicial process will be clarified for those who set administrative guidelines. Public awareness of the threats these problems pose to the economy and to society and the injustices they heap on individuals should stimulate support for those who seek solutions.

Besides administrative adjustments, there are other solutions to the problems of workers' compensation. Jobs should be designed so injuries do not occur. Prospective employees should be tested to determine that they are fit for the job and will not be injured by it and then should be retested periodically for fitness to continue with the work they are doing. People should learn in school how to protect their backs and otherwise avoid job-related injury, and job-site training should reinforce that knowledge. These are, of course, ideals that are difficult to reach when economic compromises must be made.

The other, perhaps most difficult and most important solution to workers' compensation problems is that individual people understand them. People need to understand what workers' compensation should and should not do for them, and they should be aware of the dangers that exist if they expect the wrong things. This is so important that a case history should serve to illustrate the points. This is not an unusual case. With insignificant variations related to age, sex, job detail, and local legal process, thousands of cases like Victor's occur every day.

Victor's Story

Victor was doing all right. He was 35 and thought he was in good health. He had been working at a good job for 12 years. Some of the work was and always would be physically demanding, but he had accumulated experience and skill along with it and had never been hurt. Some younger workers didn't seem to want to work as hard as he did, and sometimes he would take on more than he should to show them up. Sometimes, too, he made sudden excessive efforts out of frustration with Jenkins, the new supervisor, who seemed too demanding and did not seem to appreciate how valuable Victor's years of experience made him to the company.

Victor and Sally had three kids. Sally used to work but now stayed home to keep up with the house and the kids. Victor was tired when he got home from work, and he didn't have much time to do anything except eat and help out some with the kids. He had trouble getting around to all of the things that needed doing around the house. He bowled and did a little fishing sometimes, but he didn't have much time for exercise or recreation. He was beginning to lose some of his muscle tone, was letting his belly hang over his belt a little, and had begun to notice some stiff, aching pains in his lower back. He knew he smoked too much, but his health had been good otherwise, and he felt like he was under a lot of stress. He didn't know much about personal health care or about body mechanics and never really thought much about either.

One Friday afternoon, Victor was feeling pretty frustrated at work. Jenkins had been on them all week to get a job done. The younger guys were thinking about Friday night instead of the job. They were behind schedule. Victor was angry because the supervisor complained to him and it wasn't his fault. He was working fast and furious when the back pain hit him. He grabbed his back and fell to his knees. Someone called Jenkins, who seemed a little perturbed, told the other guys to do the heavy stuff, and told Victor to finish up as best he could. Victor limped through the rest of the shift.

That night, Victor worried about his back. He drank some beer and went to bed early. The next morning, he was a little sore but decided to go ahead with some gardening he had been putting off. He got by fairly well until he bent over and lifted a sack of fertilizer. Pain shot from his back into his hip and thigh. He felt like he couldn't straighten up. He sat down in the garden and waited until Sally and the kids helped him to bed.

On Sunday, he rested, and his back seemed a little better. He went back to work on Monday. As soon as he got there, Jenkins began pushing him to catch up on the work schedule. As he worked, he felt scared. Little twinges of back pain that he would have paid no attention to caused him to stop, hold his back, and make sure he was all right. He couldn't keep up with the work and was afraid to try harder. He talked to the supervisor, who advised him to go to the doctor.

Victor went to see Dr. Clark, his family doctor. Doctor Clark worked Victor in to a very busy schedule. When Dr. Clark heard that Victor had hurt his back at work, she didn't spend a lot of time examining him. She told him the chances were excellent that he would soon be over it, gave him some pills, and told him to go home to rest. Victor had prided himself on not missing work because of minor illness. He didn't want to go home to rest, but he knew they wouldn't let him back on the job without the doctor's approval.

Victor felt restless and nervous at home. He smoked a lot and drank a lot of beer. Sally was busy with the house and the kids and didn't have much time to care for Victor's problems. He started helping out with the housework and the kids and found that he could do most of those things without too much back pain.

Victor kept his appointment to see Dr. Clark in two weeks. Victor was still afraid of what it would be like if he went back to work. He wasn't sure his back was fine, he thought Jenkins would really push him, and he was afraid of having the back pain he had had before. He told Dr. Clark that he was still hurting. The doctor gave him an impatient look, a prescription for a different medicine, and another "not to work" slip.

Victor returned to what was getting to be a little more routine for him at home. He had begun to receive his workers' compensation checks, which were not as much as he could make working, but they made being off a little more tolerable. He began to catch up with some of the house repairs he had been putting off, and he got the garden in better shape than it had ever been in. He still had periodic twinges of back pain, but he was learning how to work around them.

Two weeks later, he told Dr. Clark that he still had periodic back pain. Dr. Clark told him he should go back to work but shouldn't do heavy lifting. She gave him a "light duty" slip, which Victor took back to his supervisor. Jenkins talked to him more than usual. He said he had been under a lot of pressure to increase productivity. He had been told that company profits were down and layoffs were threatened. He had had to train the younger guys to do the specialized, more responsible things that Victor used to do. Though he would love to have Victor back, there was really no such thing as "light duty" on this job, and union regulations would forbid putting him on some other job.

Victor felt frustrated and worried about the work situation, but his daily routine was becoming more tolerable to him. They could make it on the compensation checks for a while. He could start work on an addition to the house, which they had desperately needed but had not been able to afford to pay someone else to do. Victor was more out of shape than ever because he had been off and hadn't exercised at all, but the new project brightened his spirits. He worked hard at it in spite of some back pain, which he more or less controlled by drinking beer as he worked.

After one long day of work on the house, he went to bed early because his back was worse. The next morning, he could hardly move. He told Dr. Clark he had done a little work around home trying to get in shape to go back to his job. Dr. Clark referred him to Dr. Duncan, an orthopedic surgeon.

Dr. Duncan told Victor that the x rays showed a "degenerating disc" and that it would be best for Victor to wear a back support and to take some physical therapy. He had to go back three times each week for heat, massage, and ultrasound treatments. The physical therapist said there were "muscle spasms" in Victor's back that needed to be worked out.

Victor was getting worried. He had stopped going out with his friends for bowling or other recreation. Things were getting pretty strained between him and Sally. He was irritable and he, Sally, and the kids all seemed to be getting on one another's nerves. The compensation checks weren't really keeping up with the bills. His back still hurt.

He went back to Dr. Duncan and complained a lot about how severe his back pain was, though he knew it wasn't just the back pain that was getting to him. Dr. Duncan put him in the hospital for more therapy. Things were a little better in the hospital. It was a break from the stress at home, and at least he didn't have to look at the bills piling up. Jenkins came to see him, but the news from work was not good. They couldn't take Victor back unless he was "100 percent." Jenkins suggested that he "go on disability."

After two weeks in the hospital, Victor went home. He felt better at first, but the problems at home were still there, only worse, and when he tested his back out with some work around home, it still hurt.

He had to do something to get his bills paid, so he went back to Dr. Duncan to see about "going on disability." The doctor told Victor that it wasn't really up to him. He would cooperate by sending in a report if Victor applied, but he couldn't say that Victor was totally disabled from doing any kind of work. The social security office said that the medical reports did not suggest total disability or that there was substantial reason to assume he would be completely unable to work for more than a year, so he wasn't eligible for benefits. He could appeal if he wanted to, but they said he probably would lose the appeal.

Victor went back to Dr. Duncan and told him that he felt perfectly well, had no more back pain, and wanted to go back to his old job. Dr. Duncan thought Victor looked like he was pretty far out of shape to be doing heavy work and that his history of being out for so long with back pain made it somewhat unlikely that he could sustain his work. On the other hand, he felt sympathetic with Victor's dilemma, and he hadn't found anything seriously wrong that he would consider a danger to Victor. He gave him a "fit for work" slip and told him to be careful.

Jenkins seemed reluctant about having Victor back. Jenkins had big problems keeping ahead of things at work. He already had plugged the holes Victor had left, and he wasn't sure Victor was dependable. Regulations provided that Victor be given his job back when he was medically fit, so they would have to work it out. Victor felt like Jenkins pushed him harder than ever, and the job seemed harder than it used to be. Some of the old crew was gone, and the new ones didn't show him a lot of respect or help him out very much.

Besides all that, Victor really was out of shape. He couldn't keep up with the work, and he began to miss some days. They told him at work that they were sorry but they would have to let him go.

The adjuster for the insurance company contacted Victor and said that they would like to make a settlement. Victor didn't know anything about that, but he knew he was getting nowhere and that he needed some money to pay some debts.

He went to see Dr. Edwards, another orthopedic surgeon who was to examine him for the insurance company. Dr. Edwards was very nice to him, but told him that he couldn't really find anything wrong and that he would report that there was no permanent impairment. Victor asked him, "What about the disintegrating discs?" Dr. Edwards explained that what Victor had been told he had was a "degenerating disc" and that degeneration of a disc may be a normal process not necessarily related to pain or injury.

Victor felt desperate and didn't know what to do next. A friend suggested that he consult with Lynn Jones, an attorney. Ms. Jones seemed more sympathetic with Victor's plight than the doctors or anyone else had been. She told Victor that his situation looked bad and that the medical records really didn't document that much was wrong. She said that without medical data to support him he didn't have much of a case with either the insurance company or social security. She suggested that Victor go to another doctor. Maybe the opinion of a different specialist would help. She suggested Dr. Frazier, a neuro-surgeon.

Victor felt that none of the doctors had really appreciated how badly he had been hurting. He could go through an office exam without those awful pains he sometimes had, so they really hadn't seen his trouble. He decided that this time he should exaggerate a little bit so the doctor wouldn't think his pain didn't amount to much.

It was hard to tell from Dr. Frazier's reaction what he thought. He told Victor that he seemed to be in a lot of pain, that he had found it very hard to examine Victor, and that he could not really explain such severe pain on the basis of office findings. To be thorough, he could put Victor in the hospital to do a myelogram.

Dr. Frazier said that the myelogram showed a bulging disc. He had seen a lot worse, but it wasn't quite normal either. It could be the source of Victor's pain, but he couldn't be sure. If he surgically removed the disc, it would help to relieve the pain a lot if it had been the source of the pain, but it wouldn't help if it hadn't. He was willing to do it only if Victor was absolutely sure that his pain was severe and not being helped by any of the other treatments. Victor said that he couldn't live with things the way they were. If there was any chance at all that the operation would help, he wanted to have it.

Dr. Frazier said that the operation had gone well. The disc was bulging some, and he had removed it. He couldn't really tell from looking at it whether or not it had been the source of the pain, but he hoped for the best. He gave Victor this news in an encouraging, hopeful way. Victor felt so relieved that something finally had been done that he felt better already.

Two months later, Victor told Dr. Frazier that when he tried to go back to doing any kind of work around home his back still hurt. Dr. Frazier said that there was nothing else he could do. He suggested that Victor go back to Dr. Duncan. Dr. Duncan taught him some exercises to get him back in shape. Victor had made a brief try with back exercises when he was first taking physical therapy. He thought that it hadn't worked then and wouldn't work now. He did a few exercises but didn't try very hard or for very long.

Sally had gone back to work to try to get them out of their financial difficulties. Victor had to take over the care of the kids and the house. He managed to do those things but didn't enjoy them much. There wasn't much else in his life. He and Sally had pretty much given up their sex life through all these frustrations and because sex sometimes hurt Victor's back. He might have enjoyed trying to get back to bowling and fishing with his friends, but he felt embarrassed to be out enjoying himself when he was supposed to be so disabled that he couldn't work for a living.

Victor went back to Dr. Duncan, complaining more vigorously than ever about back pain. Dr. Duncan said that he wasn't sure anything would help. He said that Victor did have some degenerative changes in his back and that his back may have been weakened a little bit more by the disc surgery. It was possible that a fusion operation to strengthen the lower back would help, but he couldn't make any promises. Even if it helped, it might take a long time to see the result.

After the fusion operation, Victor wasn't sure whether he felt better or not. It had been so long, so many things had been said and done, and so many changes had occurred. He felt confused and uncertain about how he felt. He was afraid to do anything. He missed his job. He even missed Jenkins. Sally was off at work, and when she was home she wasn't very patient with him. He wasn't as good with the kids as she would like, and they didn't really have fun together anymore. He knew he was drinking too much. Some of the medicine he had taken after the surgery made him feel a little better, and he was still relying on that, too.

Dr. Duncan told Victor that the x rays showed the fusion was solid and that he should go back to work.

He had no work to go to.

Ms. Jones said that they would have to try to settle with the insurance company. She said that Victor would have to go to other doctors for opinions to arrive at a disability rating. Ms. Jones would have to take depositions from all of the doctors. It sounded good to Victor that he was finally going to be able to bring home some money, but it worried him that it might be a long time yet. It also worried him that Ms. Jones had warned him not to expect too much. The judgment would be based on the impairment rating, which was likely to be in the 10 to 20 percent range. Of course, the award would be reduced by the fee Ms. Jones would have to take for all of the hours of work this would be for her.

Months passed, and nothing seemed to happen. Records were slow in coming. Depositions were set way in advance to accommodate everyone's schedule and then would be canceled and set further in advance. The hearing date was pushed further and further into the future. Sally became more impatient and insisted that Victor do something. He didn't know what he could do. He asked Ms. Jones if he could go to one of the depositions.

At the deposition, Victor was dismayed to find that Ms. Jones and the attorney for the insurance company talked to each other like they were old friends. Afterwards, Ms. Jones explained to Victor that they argued cases like his almost every day and that they were friends. That didn't mean she wasn't doing everything she could to look out for Victor's interest. Victor understood that, but the whole deposition had upset him. It was all preoccupied with concerns about percentages and about the meanings of particular words, not much that seemed to be unique to the feelings that Victor had about his own problem.

Ms. Jones said that if they settled in advance of the hearing, she thought she could get the insurance company to agree to one of the higher percentage figures that had been obtained from the various doctors. When she told Victor how much money that would mean to him, Victor thought it was nowhere near what they would need to make up for what they had lost. Ms. Jones said that she realized that, but it could be even less if they didn't settle. There had been some questions raised about whether the accident at work had really caused all this trouble and whether Victor had really done all he should to care for himself. If the court accepted some of those things, he could end up with nothing but bills to pay.

Victor decided he had no choice but to accept the settlement. "What can I do now?" he asked. Ms. Jones told him he could appeal the social security decision, but she would have to charge another legal fee and they probably would lose. She knew Victor would have a hard time finding a job if he told potential employers about the history of his back problem, but it was important that he tell the truth about it or he would not be covered if any future problem did occur.

Dr. Duncan and Dr. Frazier said that there wasn't anything else they could do. They would like to help him to find work if they could, but they couldn't honestly tell an employer that he wasn't a risk for back injury.

Victor is now more out of condition than ever. He smokes, eats, drinks, and takes medicine too much. He has little sexual or recreational life. His wife is tired from working and trying to make up to the kids for what they have lost through all of this. Their financial situation has suffered, and the prospects for the future are not bright. Victor wonders, "Where did it all go wrong?"

The answer to Victor's question is not a simple one. This entire book seeks answers to that question and gives some of them.

One answer is to understand the system, to understand the dangers that lurk if you compromise your life because of back pain, and to know that some paths that may seem attractive at first can lead to disaster. You may be forced to make some compromises, but if you understand all the implications of them, you will make smart choices.

None of the characters in Victor's story is evil. None of them was dishonest. They all meant well and were trying to do their jobs. There is fault in a system that can lead to such a dreadful outcome as Victor's in spite of everyone's good intentions. Much of the problem is that each person only sees his or her part of the system and doesn't see the whole picture or even communicate very well with the others about his or her perceptions. That part of the problem can be corrected on an individual basis, and it is hoped that reading this story has encouraged you to do your share.

Who is the big loser in workers' compensation? There are no winners in Victor's story. The doctors, lawyers, and insurance people make their fees, but outcomes like Victor's do not make for satisfying work. Society and the status of the economy are losers for the reasons made obvious by the statistics cited earlier. There is no question, though, that the big losers are the people with back pain. Those with truly disabling back conditions are not justly compensated. Even bigger losers are those whose back conditions would not have been disabling had they not been led, like Victor, into difficulties so complex that it became uncertain how much was caused by the original back problem.

Whatever adjustments are made, the back pain sufferer is the one who ends up with the consequences. Long after the doctors and lawyers are paid and the insurance companies and employers have discharged what has been determined to be their responsibilities, the person with the back pain is left with the consequences. If those consequences are the loss of a good job, the loss of power in the job market, and the loss of a sense of accomplishment and fellowship from work, the price has been high for anything that may have been gained. If it leads one to forsake a path of wellness for the one of the chronic low back pain patient with all of the manifestations described throughout this text, the price certainly will have been exorbitant.

No one is in a position to look out for your interests like you are.

There are many things you can do. Try to choose work you are physically fit to do. Maintain your fitness to do your job. Work safely. Know what workers' compensation insurance will and will not do for you. If you are injured, make a real effort to return to and maintain whatever work you can do as soon as it is safe. Understand and take a long, honest look at the short- and long-term consequences of the choices you must make. Whatever the financial and social consequences of your decisions, do not pay the price of good health.

13
ANATOMY

Your lower back must provide strength to maintain an upright posture. It also must move to allow twisting, side-to-side motion, and forward-and-back bending. It protects vital structures within your abdomen and pelvis and provides safe passage for the nerves downward from the spinal cord to the legs. You expect it to do all of this without pain, over a lifetime of stresses.

Details of how stress affects the structure of the back, how the back is constructed to withstand those stresses, and how those stresses are distributed through the back are still being discovered. The anatomical structure, the chemical makeup, and the effects of stress and movement are all different for different people. They all change every day through one person's lifetime and even undergo cyclic changes within the same day. Advances in technology and understanding are constantly providing new ways to look at the structures, determine the chemical composition, or apply engineering principles to analysis of the movements and stresses. With so many different ways to look at so many different things, all of which change all the time, it is not hard to understand that mysteries of the structure and workings of the back are still waiting to be discovered.

The scaffold upon which the low back is built is composed of interconnected segments of bone. Living bone is not a china- or ivory-like substance as it appears in museum specimens. Living bone is composed of fibers made of collagen, which is a protein. The fibers are woven and stranded together and laced with deposits of crystals of calcium and other minerals. In the thick outer cortex, the collagen fibers are densely packed together. In the thinner, lacier marrow portions of bone, they are more loosely packed. Blood flows through the bone and provides oxygen and minerals that sustain living bone cells and allow the crystals to reform themselves, maintaining strength and balance.

The bones are bound together by ligaments. Ligaments are rope-like structures composed of fibers of collagen woven and stranded together. They anchor into the bone by intimately bonding and inter-weaving with the collagen structure of the bone. The ligaments in their normal state do not contain mineral crystals, though bone or calcium deposits may form in them as a result of injury repair or repeated stress.

Most ligaments, like a woven rope, have some slack built into the weave but little true elasticity. They serve as check reins against excessive motion of the bones, and they maintain the bones in their normal relationship to one another.

The places where bones interconnect are called joints. Joints vary greatly in shape, composition, and function. The back contains some unique joints that are quite different from one another and have some features unlike the joints in the arms and legs.

Each separate bone of the lower spine is called a lumbar vertebra. In most people, there are five of these. Above them are the 12 thoracic vertebrae, which are separate, interconnected vertebrae much like the lumbar vertebrae except that they have ribs attached to them. The lumbar vertebra connect below to the sacrum, which is the solid base of the spine. The sacrum is much larger than any one lumbar vertebra. Large, barely movable joints (sacroiliac joints) anchor the sacrum to the pelvis. The pelvis bones and the sacrum are bound together so tightly that they move together. Together they form the stable platform upon which the movable spine is balanced.

Every two adjacent lumbar vertebrae make direct contact on the posterior (back) side by a paired set of joints—the facet joints. In front, they make contact and are supported by a complex, specialized joint called the intervertebral disc.

The vertebrae are numbered, starting with the highest lumbar vertebra, lumbar 1 or L1, down to the lowest, lumbar 5 or L5. The sacrum frequently is designated S1 when reference is made to the top part of the sacrum.

The combination of two adjacent vertebrae connected by a pair of facet joints and a disc is called a segment of the spine. The segments and the discs they include are designated by naming the two vertebrae, such as L3–L4 or L3–4. The lowest disc, L5–S1, is also sometimes called the lumbosacral disc. Not all people have five lumbar vertebrae; thus, the lumbosacral segment in some instances is L4–S1 or L6–S1.

Each vertebra forms a ring of bone around a central space. (See Figure 13.) When the vertebrae are locked together by the joints, the spaces line up, forming a tunnel or canal called the vertebral canal. In the thoracic spine, the canal is filled by the spinal cord, the cerebrospinal fluid that surrounds it, and a membrane sac (meninges) that holds the fluid. The spinal cord ends in the upper lumbar area, but the sac full of spinal fluid continues through the canal of the lumbar spine and sacrum. The roots of the spinal nerves on their way to the pelvis and the legs pass through this fluid-filled sac. At each vertebral segment, one pair of nerves comes out of the sac, passes through the vertebral canal, and then exits through spaces between the side walls of the vertebrae.

The distance the nerve travels after leaving the sac until it leaves the vertebral canal is quite short. The nerve takes that short course along the anterior and lateral corner of the vertebral canal in a groove called the lateral recess. The spaces between the vertebrae through which the nerves pass are called foramina, each one being called a foramen or an intervertebral foramen.

After the nerves exit through the foramina, many of them join

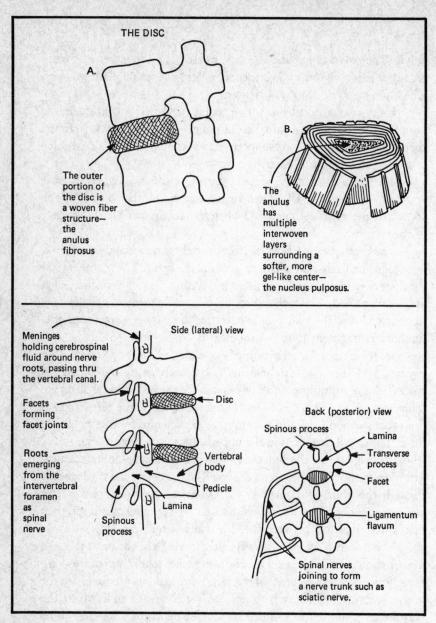

FIGURE 13. Lumbar Spine Anatomy.

together to form trunks that pass down, giving branches to muscles and bringing back sensory information. The largest of these trunks is the sciatic nerve, which courses through the buttock and down the leg. You may visualize the sciatic nerve as an upside-down tree, which originates from roots from the lower back, forms a large trunk, and gradually divides into branches as it passes down the leg.

Besides the ligaments that hold the vertebrae together at their joints, additional ligaments pass from one vertebra to the next and from pelvis to vertebrae, attaching at connecting points on the vertebrae called processes. These are guy wires and check reins and cannot actively control the movement of the spine.

The active control of movement, the fine-tuning of posture, and the protection of the spine from excessive stress are the jobs of the muscles. The vertebrae have muscle attachments on all sides. Muscles of various thicknesses and lengths pass in all directions. The muscles function for the lumbar spine by direct attachment to the lumbar vertebrae and indirectly by pressure exerted through the abdominal contents and by positioning the chest, hips, and pelvis.

We know that muscle weakness, muscle stiffness, and loss of muscle function are very important contributors to back pain. Doctors are often not able to zero in on one spot in one muscle to locate the source of pain. Most likely, back trouble doesn't happen that way very often. Also, the diagnostic means to pinpoint muscle problems accurately aren't available.

The same difficulty with precision applies to most ligament problems. Many ligaments function in different ways, under different circumstances, and in intimate relationships to the muscles around them. One single point in one single ligament will not often be likely, by itself, to cause persisting back pain. Even if such a cause were likely, the diagnostic means to prove it is not available.

Doctors can be reasonably accurate in saying that a back condition is related to muscle or ligament problems. However, they cannot often pinpoint precisely a ligament or muscle, find exactly what is wrong with it, and determine how long it is going to take it to recover.

Some common causes of back pain often do lend themselves to very precise identification. Many of those involve abnormalities that occur in the intervertebral disc.

The intervertebral disc is a complicated anatomic structure. (See Figure 13.) Though its overall shape may be somewhat like a tiddly-wink, its makeup is anything but a single, predictable material.

The disc is located between the top of the body of one vertebra and the bottom of the body of the vertebra above it. The body of the vertebra is the largest part of the vertebra, and it is located in the front (anterior) portion of the spine. The back of the vertebral body makes up the front wall of the vertebral canal. The body is somewhat like a baked biscuit in that all of the outside surface of it is thicker, more densely packed bone, whereas the center marrow portion is spongier.

The outermost portion of the disc is a ligament, passing from the edges of the hard, peripheral rim of the body above to that below. It forms a complete ring. It is a multilayered, woven structure composed somewhat like the tough weave of an automobile tire. The fibers blend with crystal-laden fibers of the bone above and below. This ring of ligament, completely surrounding the space between two adjacent vertebral bodies, is called the anulus fibrosus. It is a very tough structure which, for most people, survives a lifetime of extraordinary stresses.

The center of each disc is called the nucleus pulposus. Its chemical content and even its gross physical properties change throughout life and even vary within a single day. Its molecules have a high capacity to attract and hold water. They form a gel-like substance.

The central nucleus pulposus and the surrounding rim of anulus fibrosus do not have a distinct border between them as in, say, a jelly donut. They gradually blend together. The outer layers of anulus are almost all tough, dense collagen fibers. The inner layers contain some of the gel-like molecules. Some collagen fibers extend in toward the centers so that there are some fibers throughout, though generally, the closer to the center, the smaller the number of fibers.

The nucleus pulposus is held by walls of anulus fibrosus and by a ceiling and floor composed of the bone of the vertebral bodies above and below. This portion of the bone of the body is called the chondral plate or end plate. The chondral plate is covered on the side of the nucleus by cartilage, the smooth, less brittle material you observe on joint surfaces at the ends of bones.

The inner part of the adult intervertebral disc has no blood flow. The disc is the largest avascular structure in the human body. The water exchange and chemical transformations that occur in the center of the discs take place by diffusion through the chondral plates and outer portions of the anulus.

The content of the nucleus changes throughout life. It gradually loses its capacity to hold water and becomes less gel-like and more fibrous. Although this is a normal life process, this change is called degeneration of the disc.

The nucleus of an adolescent or a young adult may be about the consistency of a raw oyster, the nucleus of middle age is like a boiled shrimp, and in older people the nucleus becomes more gristly.

The water content of a young, healthy nucleus pulposus may be as high as 88 percent. The disc will follow some of the physical properties of a liquid. One is Pascal's Law, written in the seventeenth century. The law states that a force anywhere on a contained liquid is transmitted undiminished throughout that liquid. This explains why the disc can act as a good shock absorber, keeping the vertebrae apart and the anulus ligaments taut. You also can see that if the container has a weakened area, forces will continue to be exerted against it as long as the nucleus remains liquid and remains contained.

As discs lose their water content, they become smaller. This allows the vertebrae to settle closer together. Discs actually lose some water content through the day and replenish it at night, so if you measure very accurately, you will observe that you are slightly shorter in the evening than you are in the morning. The disc is a little swollen in the morning compared to its state later in the day. The water content is almost but not entirely replaced at night, so that very slowly over a lifetime the discs lose volume. That is one reason why people become shorter as they age.

As aging and loss of water from the discs occur, the nucleus behaves less like a liquid. It may form lobules, or compartments that behave hydrostatically in part and in part more like a solid. Those changes diminish the discs' normal shock-absorbing function. They may be beneficial changes, however, in cases where a protruding nucleus is exerting pressure on a weak spot in the anulus.

All discs degenerate. That much is normal. For some people, one or more discs may degenerate long before their other discs or at a younger age than for other people. This early or rapid degeneration of a disc is sometimes, though not most often, explained by specific injury. Degeneration sometimes, though not often, is associated with pain or other symptoms. Many times, evidence of degeneration is observed on x rays taken for reasons other than back pain.

Vertebral Canal, Lateral Recesses, and Foramina

The posterior roof of the vertebral canal is formed by bony parts of the vertebra called laminae and the central backward protruding spinous process. The spinous processes can be seen and felt through the skin of thin people. The laminae are more narrow than the body of the vertebra, so there are spaces between the back sides of the adjacent vertebrae. These spaces are occupied by ligaments of unusual elasticity, the yellow ligaments or ligamenta flava.

At the outer corner of the vertebral canal, where the laminae that form the roof meet the pedicles that form the side walls, processes protrude up and down on both sides of each vertebra. These processes are the facets. They join with the facets of adjacent vertebrae like clasped hands, forming the facet joints.

The side wall pedicles join the large, anterior portion of the vertebra, the body. The bodies and the discs that lie between them comprise the anterior wall or floor of the vertebral canal.

The foramina are along the sides of the vertebral canal. The foramen is formed in front by the vertebral body and disc. It is formed above and below by the pedicles and in back by the facets.

The lower lumbar vertebral canal may be trefoil-shaped, similar to the configuration created by holding three pencils together. The widest portion is across the floor of the canal, over the bodies and discs. The trefoil is created by the facets, which take up space in the upper corners of the canal. The spaces in the lower corners under the facets are called the lateral recesses.

Settling together of vertebrae that occurs as a result of disc degeneration causes some decrease in the spaces between the vertebrae. The foramina get smaller. For most people, this never matters. Most foramina are about the size of a thumb, so that even if the size of the foramen diminishes, there is usually plenty of room left for the nerve. The nerve is usually smaller than a pencil.

The lateral recesses are generally smaller than the foramina. Some people have large, triangular-shaped vertebral canals, so their lateral recesses are not well defined. Others have small vertebral canals with narrow, well-defined lateral recesses. Disc bulging, bone spurs in the anulus, facet overlap, and facet spurs may narrow the lateral recesses. For people with small canals and well-defined lateral recesses, that narrowing may lead to a pinched nerve root.

Stenosis means a narrowing of the passageway. In the lumbar spine, stenosis may refer to narrowing of the vertebral canal, narrowing of the lateral recess, or narrowing of the foramen. Symptoms depend upon the location and degree of the stenosis.

Bad Discs

In the short course the spinal nerve takes between the meningeal sac and the foramen, the nerve passes right next to or over an intervertebral disc. Nerve roots, especially the fifth lumbar and first sacral, are more vulnerable in this short segment than any other nerves in the body. At least, more people experience pain and dysfunction because of trouble in this segment of nerve than because of any other problem caused by peripheral nerve disorders.

The woven fibers of anulus, tough as they are, sometimes tear or pull loose at a portion of their moorings into the vertebral body. The tremendous pressures inside the nucleus exert forces against the weak spot. The body's attempts to repair tears of the anulus fibers are slow and may be obstructed by repeated stresses.

The nucleus material may move gradually into the weak area and cause the anulus to bulge out. A blister-like enlargement on the surface of the disc may form. If the nucleus has begun to degenerate, this bulged-out portion may contain fragments of nucleus that have dried and separated from the gel-like portion of the normal nucleus.

The disc may bulge out in any direction, even into the bone above or below. It is unfortunate, however, that the place where it bulges most often is right under or next to the nerve roots.

The disc between the fourth and fifth lumbar vertebrae and the one between the fifth lumbar and the sacrum are the ones most likely to cause trouble. These discs cushion vertebrae that do not sit directly on top of each other. They must resist the weight that is brought down through the spine and also the shear stress that tends to make the vertebra above slide down the vertebra below. This shear stress can be diminished by tilting your pelvis to make the base—the sacrum—more flat. If the angle of the sacrum is 30 degrees, the shear stress may be calculated mathematically to be about half the weight transmitted through the disc. If it is increased to 50 degrees, the shear stress increases to about 75 percent of that weight. Reducing shear stress, therefore, is one of the benefits of decreasing your lordosis.

Bulging of the anulus and movement of nucleus material into the area of the bulge, like a tire tube with a blistered area, pose the threat of a blowout or rupture. If this occurs, the fragment of nucleus may move out into the vertebral canal. The pain pattern then may change, depending on where and how the nerve is irritated.

The movement of nucleus material into the canal, whether by a bulge or a rupture, diminishes the size of the canal and crowds the nerve root. Depending on the size of the canal at the spot to begin with and the size of the disc fragment, it may narrow it enough to pinch the nerve.

Experiments have shown that simply pinching a nerve root usually does not cause all of the symptoms people have from bad discs. Some of the chemicals involved in the degeneration process of the nucleus may escape and irritate the nerve. The body's attempt to repair the anulus may cause inflammation and scarring of the nerve. Some of the symptoms may come from small branches of the nerve in the area rather than from pressure on the large nerve root. People who have many symptoms are likely to have some combination of these factors.

The practice of explaining symptoms by identifying the site of difficulty is not an exact science. The source of certain pain patterns and patterns of nerve dysfunction can be traced to this area where the disc is in proximity to the nerve root with more precision than can the sources of other common back disorders. When these specific patterns of pain and dysfunction exist, those who are experienced in evaluating these disorders can predict with a high degree of accuracy the spot of origin of the trouble. This accuracy can be improved further by using x-ray techniques. The most widely used technique, the myelogram, requires placing contrast material (dye) into the spinal fluid outlining the vertebral canal. Disc bulging or rupture usually will be seen as a failure of formation of the full outline of the canal.

Spondylolysis and Spondylolisthesis

Some people have weak areas in the vertebrae where the laminae branch out above and below to form the facets. This area is called the pars interarticularis. These defects occur in about 5 percent of American whites and a little less often in blacks. They are called spondylolysis. In most people, they cause little or no trouble. In some, they cause pain. Sometimes they are associated with forward slippage of the front part of the vertebra. Slippage of one vertebra forward on another is called spondylolisthesis. Spondylolisthesis may occur because of spondylolysis or for several other reasons. Spondylolisthesis and spondylolysis are not necessarily associated with symptoms.

Spondylosis and Spondylitis

The combination of disc degeneration and bone thickening with spur formation is sometimes called spondylosis. Spondylosis occurs to some extent in everyone and usually is not symptomatic. The normal smooth gliding of the facet joints is sometimes lost because of spondylosis. Spondylitis is a general term that refers to any of many different kinds of arthritis that may affect the spine.

Surgery

By far the most common operation done on the lower back is for removal of a bad disc. The operation frequently has been called laminectomy because some or all of the lamina usually is removed to get to the disc. Unless the whole lamina is removed, the term is not precise, but it is still in common use. The more precise terms laminotomy or hemi-laminotomy also are often used. All of these terms refer more to how the surgeon gets there than to what is done. If a portion of a disc is removed, the operation may be called a discectomy.

Most disc surgery is done through a midline incision. Once through the skin and fat, the surgeon moves to one side of the spinous process and lamina, pulling the muscles back from the bone. Some ligamentum flavum and some bone are removed to provide access to the vertebral canal. If fragments of nucleus pulposus are found loose in the canal, they are removed. If the disc is found to be abnormal but the nucleus is still held close to the disc space by stretched-out remnants of anulus fibrosus, the surgeon opens the enclosure and removes the bad part of the nucleus.

Most of the strength and function of the disc is provided by the anulus fibrosus. Except for sometimes making a small cut in it, the surgeon seldom disturbs the anulus during ordinary disc surgery. The loose and offending fragments of nucleus are removed, but since there is usually still some good nucleus blending with the anulus, the surgeon seldom attempts to remove all of the nucleus. By no means, then, in ordinary disc surgery, is the whole disc removed. Therefore, there is seldom any need to replace what was removed. Nature fills the void with scar tissue and sometimes by slight settling together of the vertebral bodies.

In certain selected cases, the nucleus can be removed by chemonucleolysis. For that technique, an enzyme is injected through a needle into the disc. The enzyme causes a portion of the disc to dissolve. The net result may be about the same as surgery.

Another common operation done on the lower back is a fusion, also sometimes called an arthrodesis. The usual reason for having a fusion is that one of the segments of the spine is unstable. Criteria of stability are not precise. If there is abnormal motion that has produced deformity or threatens to do so, or if there is motion that is the source of pain, then a fusion may be suggested.

Most fusions are done by roughening the bone on either side of the site of abnormal or painful motion and then placing a bone graft over the roughened areas. The bone graft is most often taken from the back of the pelvic bone, near the site of the low back abnormality. Sometimes wires, screws, or rods are used internally to hold the segment still while the bone graft takes. Such internal fixation is not always necessary.

A fusion results in loss of motion in the segment that is fused. Motion above and below may increase or, at least, the stresses above and below may increase, so a fusion is apt to relieve pain only when the trouble was isolated to the segment that was fused.

Understanding the anatomy of the back pain has led surgeons to be able to help many people with back pain. Most back problems, however, would not be relieved by surgery. Those who are helped by surgery are only helped, not cured. No back operation leaves a completely normal back. Understanding and proper application of the principles of back care as discussed elsewhere in this book are essential to obtain and maintain a healthy back.

14
OTHER CAUSES
OF BACK PAIN

Most back pain is caused by injuries, wear and tear, or excessive stress. A small percentage of back pain results from specific structural abnormalities of bone, medical diseases that involve the spine, or diseases of nonstructural organs near the spine.

Scoliosis

Lateral (sideways) curvature of the spine is called scoliosis. Temporary scoliosis may result from muscle spasm. Permanent scoliosis results from a variety of injuries, diseases, and birth defects. The most common type is an inherited characteristic that appears during preadolescent and adolescent years of rapid growth.

Scoliosis is a complex problem. It is discussed here only as it relates to back pain. Deformity and functional impairment are the main worries with scoliosis. Pain is usually a relatively minor part of the problem.

Scoliosis is measured in degrees of angulation, with 0 degrees signifying a perfectly straight spine and 90 degrees meaning a right-angle bend. Less than 10 degrees is considered under most circumstances to be normal. About 5 percent of people have curvatures of more than 10 degrees. Whether or not those 5 percent have more back pain than other people has been a controversial subject.

Most information supports the opinion that back pain does not occur any more frequently among people with scoliosis than among those with straight spines. In spite of that, many authorities believe that certain individuals with scoliosis, particularly those with curvatures of more than 50 degrees, are more likely to experience severe back pain. Prevention and correction of deformity of the growing spine are the usual reasons for surgery for scoliosis. Relief from low back pain in the adult with severe lumbar scoliosis is a rare indication for surgery.

Tail Bone Pain

The tail bone, or coccyx, is located at the tip of the spine, below where most people experience back pain. Disorders of the tail bone seldom cause low back pain, but pain in the coccyx is common enough that the two often coexist.

The coccyx is composed of four or five separate bones held tightly together by ligaments. In most people, the coccyx forms a gentle forward curve. The coccyx has no important function.

A painful tail bone, called coccydynia, usually has no clearly defined cause. It sometimes follows a fracture of one of the coccyx bones, a fall on the area, or childbirth.

Tumors, infections, or other serious diseases of the coccyx are very rare. Pain in the coccyx usually can be distinguished from rectal pain because tenderness is well localized to the coccyx and bleeding or other signs of abnormality of the rectum are absent.

If you have coccydynia, you will do best to sit on a hard surface and lean forward so your weight is on your thighs. Coccydynia is a nuisance, but the pain is seldom severe. The problem usually disappears without treatment, but it may last for months. Surgery to remove the coccyx was once popular but is seldom performed now because it was not found to be reliable in relieving the pain and because most people get over coccydynia without treatment.

Hip Disorders

Abnormalities of the hip joint may coexist with back disorders. Trouble in the hip may produce pain that is mistakenly interpreted as coming from the back.

Many people refer to the upper buttock near the base of the spine as their hip. Pain in that region is more likely to be from the back than from the hip joint.

Pain from the hip joint usually is felt in the groin and sometimes down the front of the thigh to the knee. It is often aggravated by rotating the hip while sitting or lying with the knee bent.

Pain at the site of the hip may be from trochanteric bursitis or tendinitis. The greater trochanter is the large bony knob at the side of your hip just below your waist. The tendons of the powerful buttock muscles attach to the thigh bone at the greater trochanter. The wide tendon of the iliotibial band passes over the trochanter. Movement of your hip under the band is lubricated by a filmy sac—the trochanteric bursa.

Inflammation of the tendon insertion into the greater trochanter or of the trochanteric bursa will cause pain along the side of the hip. Bursitis may be acute, severe, and accompanied by exquisite tenderness over the region. Tendinitis is usually slower in coming on, more persistent, and tender only to deep pressure. Either condition may coexist with back disorders. Corticosteroid injections usually relieve the pain from bursitis and often help with tendinitis.

Tumors and Infections of the Spine

Chronic pain is reason for concern about cancer and other destructive diseases. However, since about 80 percent of people experience significant pain at some time, it is obvious that only a tiny fraction of people with back pain have tumors or infections in their spines.

Most people who have a destructive process, such as a tumor or an infection, have symptoms other than pain—unexplained weight loss, fever, loss of energy, or symptoms of dysfunction of other body organs. The pains from tumors or infections are usually persistent, unrelated to physical stress, and often worse at night. People who do not have such symptoms, especially if they have passed a medical examination, can be reasonably assured that their back pain is from a benign, nondestructive source.

Osteoporosis

Bone crystals continuously lose and replace calcium and other minerals. Many adults lose bone minerals faster than they replace them. The result is weakened bones, a condition called osteoporosis.

There are many causes of osteoporosis. The common type is unrelated to other disease, progresses most rapidly in women after menopause, and tends to get worse with aging.

Uncomplicated osteoporosis probably doesn't produce pain. Complications, however, are frequent. Fractures of the weakened bones of the spine produce back pain. Sometimes the fractures cause partial collapse of the vertebral body so that the x-ray appearance of the body is that it has been compressed, flattened down like a crushed biscuit. Other times, the fractures are tiny cracks or dents that are not visible with x rays. Osteoporotic spine fractures hurt for a while, heal and quit hurting, and then may occur again at a different site.

Compression of vertebral bodies changes the shape and appearance of the spine. Compression of one side of a vertebral body may produce scoliosis. More often, the forward bend of the spine—kyphosis—is accentuated. Increased kyphosis produces a stooped-over, shortened posture and a "dowager's hump" of the upper dorsal area. Crushing of several vertebral bodies may result in considerable loss of height.

Osteoporosis is more preventable than it is curable. Regular exercise, a calcium-rich diet, multiple vitamin and mineral diet supplements, and, under certain circumstances, hormones and/or fluoride treatments help prevent progression of osteoporosis. Treatment of back pain from osteoporosis is similar to treatment for other back pains. Time, patience, and good body mechanics are especially important while osteoporotic spine fractures are healing.

Arthritis

Osteoarthritis, the common wear-and-tear form of arthritis, produces changes in the lower back that are indistinguishable from normal changes of aging. People who have osteoarthritis in their fingers, hips, knees, or other joints at a young age may be more likely to have symptoms from similar changes in their lumbar spine.

Rheumatoid arthritis, the most common of the destructive, progressive, crippling arthridites, seldom produces low back pain. It is usual for the hip joints and the cervical spine to be crippled by rheumatoid arthritis, but for unknown reasons the lumbar spine is usually spared.

There is a group of arthritic diseases called spondyloarthropathies, a word that refers to disease of spinal joints. Included are arthritic manifestations of such general diseases as psoriasis, ulcerative colitis, and Reiter's syndrome. The most common of the spondyloarthropathies is ankylosing spondylitis.

Ankylosing spondylitis is also known, from the names of the doctors who described it, as Marie-Strumpell's disease. It has also sometimes been called rheumatoid spondylitis, an unfortunate term because the disease is completely different from rheumatoid arthritis.

Ankylosing spondylitis does not produce definite x-ray changes until the disease is well established. It was once uncommon for the diagnosis to be made until the disease had been present for years. Now, because of a blood test and better understanding of early manifestations of the disease, the diagnosis may be made sooner.

Ankylosing spondylitis is more common and more damaging for men than for women. The sacroiliac joint (where the lower spine articulates with the pelvis) and the joints of the spine are affected first. Symptoms usually begin in the second or third decade of life. Stiffness and pain, usually worse in the early mornings, are the dominant symptoms. Pain is also present in the dorsal spine more often than it is with other low back disorders.

The blood test for ankylosing spondylitis is called an HLA–B27 antigen. The test was derived from the experimental work done for tissue typing for transplant surgery. A positive test means there is a particular gene configuration on a chromosome. It is either present or absent, depending on the genetic makeup of the individual, and it will not change with symptoms.

The HLA–B27 antigen test is not specific for ankylosing spondylitis. About 5 percent of the population is HLA–B27 antigen positive. Less than 1 percent of the population has ankylosing spondylitis. Other forms of spondylolyarthropathies also occur more frequently in HLA–B27 positive people. About 95 percent of white people with ankylosing spondylitis are HLA–B27 positive; the correlation is not that high for black people.

So, not everyone who has ankylosing spondylitis is HLA–B27 positive, ankylosing spondylitis is not the only disease that occurs more often in HLA–B27 positive people, and only about 20 percent of HLA–B27 positive people have ankylosing spondylitis. In spite of these limitations, the test statistics can be correlated with signs and symptoms to result in a reasonably accurate bet about the presence or absence of this disease. Such a judgment may be very important because the symptoms of ankylosing spondylitis sometimes can mimic surgically remediable back disorders. Ankylosing spondylitis is not helped by surgery. It is helped by anti-inflammatory medicines.

Systemic lupus erythematosis is a chronic inflammatory disease of unknown origin. Lupus affects many different organs including muscles and joints. It occurs more frequently in young women. Fever, rash, sensitivity to light, pleurisy, and abnormalities of blood and urine tests usually identify this as a systemic disease, so it is not often confused with ordinary back and joint pains.

Polymyalgia rheumatica is an unusual disease which occurs in people over 50, more often in women. Severe persistent aching pain across the shoulders and buttocks are accompanied by low grade fever and a feeling of illness. It often accompanies an inflammation of the temporal arteries which run along the side of the head. The blood sedimentation rate is markedly elevated. Polymyositis is a disease which results in inflammation of muscles. There are many other unusual diseases of muscle and connective tissue which are rare causes of back pain.

The term "fibrositis syndrome" refers to the occurrence of multiple tender areas, mostly over the upper and lower back. The syndrome may be associated with emotional tensions, lack of exercise, fatigue, and sleep disorders. It is not associated with any known disease and should not be confused with potentially destructive arthritic diseases such as those discussed above.

Kidney Disease

Poorly understood back pain was once commonly attributed to kidney trouble. Patent medicines often were marketed to cure back pain by treating the kidneys. The medicines didn't help the kidneys. Very few back pains have anything to do with kidneys.

Kidney stones may produce severe back pain, especially if they become lodged in the ureter. The pain is so acute, severe, and distinguished by its recurrent waves that it is not likely to be confused with ordinary back pain. Likewise, the severe pain in the upper flank with fever and feelings of general illness that occur because of acute kidney infection are not likely to be confused with other types of lower back pain.

Chronic kidney infections, tumors, and cysts are rare causes of back pain. The pain is likely to be higher in the back than ordinary low back pain, not related to physical stress, and not relieved by rest.

Pelvic Disease

Bladder infections may produce pelvic discomfort and some low back pain. They usually also produce fever, bloody urine, pain with urination, or a feeling of illness. Men may have similar symptoms from prostate infections. The pains are so different from structural low back pain and the other symptoms are so characteristic that it is very unusual for these infections and musculoskeletal back disorders to be confused.

Fibroid tumors, endometriosis, and other disorders of the female reproductive organs may produce aching pains in the lower back. Back pain that occurs in cycle with menstrual periods may be from such pelvic abnormalities. Back pain from spinal disorders such as bulging discs also may be accentuated during menstrual periods, so cyclic pain cannot be assumed to be caused by abnormal pelvic organs.

Even though causal relationships between pelvic organ disorders and back pain cannot be assumed, women with persistent back pain should have a pelvic examination. Certainly, women with bleeding between periods, increased pain during periods, abnormal vaginal discharges, pelvic pain, or painful intercourse should have a pelvic examination.

Gastrointestinal Diseases

Cancer of the stomach, pancreas, liver, and bowel may produce back pain. The pain is usually constant, worse at night or at rest, and unrelated to body position. It is usually accompanied by weight loss, loss of energy, feelings of general illness, or symptoms of bleeding or other abnormalities of bowel function.

Ulcers of the stomach and upper bowel also may cause back pain. Usually, ulcers cause heartburn, abdominal pain, and symptoms related to food and drink intake.

Bleeding from the bowels, change in size of stools or bowel habits, jaundice, abdominal pain, nausea and vomiting, and weight loss are symptoms that demand medical evaluation and treatment. They are not symptoms of ordinary back pain and must not be ignored while treating back pain.

Circulation Problems

Blood from the heart flows to the legs through a large artery, the aorta. The aorta divides in the pelvis into right and left iliac arteries which subsequently divide into smaller arteries which go to the pelvis, buttocks, and legs.

A weak area in the wall of the aorta may be stretched out by the pressure of the contained blood. A sacular enlargement called an aneurysm may form. Abdominal aneurysms may cause back pain.

Placques of atherosclerosis or an aneurysm may decrease the blood flow into the buttock or leg muscles and can cause pain. The pain caused by reduced blood flow to large muscles occurs when those muscles are exercised. Buttock and leg pain which occurs from muscular effort may be similar to leg pains from sciatic nerve root irritation.

Pain from inadequate blood flow to leg muscles usually occurs after a predictable amount of exercise, such as walking a certain distance. The pain is often manifested as a cramp in the muscle. In contrast to pain from pinched nerves, a very brief rest of a minute or two usually completely relieves the pain from inadequate circulation.

15

PROFESSIONAL TREATMENT OF BACK PAIN

Scientific and Nonscientific Treatments

If you have read Chapter 13 on back anatomy, you have a better understanding of the medically important anatomical facts about the lumbar region than anyone did until about 50 years ago. For a treatment method to be considered to have a scientific basis, its effects must be explainable by reliable knowledge about what has gone wrong with the anatomy and chemistry to create the condition that is under treatment. Until the early 1930s, none of the common conditions that cause back pain were understood in that way.

For a treatment to be considered scientific, it must make sense; that is, it must be consistent with an adequate number of known facts. It also must be proven by well-controlled, scientific trials that the treatment method works for the reasons predicted from the knowledge of those facts. The requirement that the treatment works for the reason it is supposed to work is much more difficult to prove than you might suppose. The main reason is the very complex, many-faceted nature of back pain. All of those facets may be important regardless of the underlying cause of the pain. All of those facets must be evaluated, understood, or balanced in order to control their influence on the effect of one treatment on one disorder. Without such control there is no way of knowing whether the treatment really worked for the predicted reasons.

Another major problem is uncertainty about the underlying cause of the pain. In the past 50 years, we have proven that certain abnormalities, such as rupture of an intervertebral disc, definitely can be a source of back and sciatic pain. We also know, however, that most people with back pain don't have such a clearly demonstrable cause for the pain. We know that some people with ruptured discs don't have pain. And we know that a disc isn't always either ruptured or normal, like a light is on or off. It is more like a light controlled by a rheostat, where any shade from almost entirely normal to almost totally ruptured may be present. These facts make it very difficult to know that each individual patient treated by a certain method has the condition for which the treatment is supposed to work.

Treatments for back pain are difficult to test in the laboratory because back pain is uniquely human. Medical progress in other fields has been hastened vastly because of scientific experimentation on laboratory animals. Animal study has made a contribution to the back pain problem, but it is a rather small one. The stresses of erect posture and the anatomy of the human back don't have close counterparts in animals. Experimentation on human volunteers is limited for humane reasons and slow for legal reasons. In spite of those limitations, volunteer patients have made huge contributions to the proof that certain treatments, when applied to well-defined conditions, really are effective.

In order, then, to consider a treatment predictable and effective, we must understand what it does and we must have proof that it really does work for the reasons we understand. We have only two scientifically validated treatments for any of the common forms of back pain that meet those requirements—surgical excision of a ruptured intervertebral disc and chemonucleolysis for a ruptured intervertebral disc. Those treatments, especially in the case of surgery, were understood and thought to be effective long before they were ever proven so. They are effective for only a small minority of people who suffer from back pain. They are, however, effective for the majority of those who definitely have a ruptured intervertebral disc.

Long before there was good scientific evidence that surgical treatment was successful, there were surgeons who were certain of it. Thousands of patients gave testimony to the effectiveness of their surgery. That is not science, though, and it is not proof. Similar claims and testimonials have turned out more often to be wrong than right when subjected to the scrutiny of scientific investigation. For most treatments, such scientific investigations are never undertaken. Most unproven treatments fail the test of time and cease to be offered or requested. Many, such as the first aid measures offered in Chapter 1 of this book, persist because they make good sense in the light of known facts. Others, such as manipulation, seem to survive on the basis of testimonials.

Just because a treatment method has not been proven scientifically does not mean it will not succeed in individual cases. Some methods would stand up under scientific scrutiny but have just not been tested in the correct way. Others are effective in individual cases even if they make no sense. There is still much art in healing and in being healed. Those who work with methods they believe to be scientific don't discourage, and certainly don't deny, the effectiveness of unscientific methods. The difference is that scientifically validated methods have a more predictable result. Their effects are similar when applied for the same problem by different healers to different sufferers.

If you are going to take risks to relieve your back pain, you want to know the chance of success. Methods that have been subjected to scientific testing offer you that sort of information. Of course, the greater the risk, the more certain you want to be. Taking risks with your health from operations, drugs, or dangerous devices must be carefully weighed against potential benefits. Risking your time and financial resources are also important considerations. Time-consuming, inconvenient, and expensive treatment methods should offer more certainty of positive effect than simpler ones.

When you must rely upon testimonials and conflicting opinions about effectiveness, it is hard to make choices about treatments. When there is a lot of uncertainty, it is best to rely upon what seems reasonable, safe, and simple. Simple, as you found in Chapter 11, is not always the same as easy. Most often, it is the same as accessible, inexpensive, and safe. It most often means that you can apply the method yourself and do not have to rely on a professional.

When you do need a professional and when you feel you must accept more risk in hope of relief, you want the best science has to offer. You don't want to rely on testimonials, media-sensationalized new methods, and marketing gimmicks. Often, the best science has to offer is what makes the most sense in the light of currently available known facts. In two instances—surgery and chemonucleolysis for ruptured discs—it can offer more.

Surgery for Sciatica from Ruptured Discs

The usual reason why people have intervertebral discs surgically removed is to relieve pain. The type of pain for which this treatment is most reliable is sciatic pain.

Sciatic pain—sciatica—usually feels like it comes out of the lower back or buttock and radiates down the back of the leg to below the knee. Sciatic pain usually is aggravated by position changes that either stretch the nerve or cause increase in pressure around the roots of the nerve. The pain usually is sharp or electrical in feeling. Not all pains that radiate down the leg are sciatica.

Pains that come from sciatic irritation are not the same for everyone. For the same person, the type of pain may vary from time to time. It is difficult for the sufferer to localize and characterize pains in a way that defines whether or not the pain is sciatica. It may be difficult for a professional to make that distinction. It is so important because many, though not all, patients with sciatica have ruptured discs as the source of their trouble. It is for relief of this specific symptom of sciatica in those specific patients—those with ruptured intervertebral discs—that surgical removal of the disc is of proven effectiveness.

Sciatica has afflicted people and attracted the attention of healers since ancient times. Hippocrates described it but erroneously called it "affection of the crural vein." Cato used the word *ischiados,* which refers to the origin of the pain from the back of the hip and gives a clue to the source of the term *sciatica.* The term has come through English and other western languages in many forms: *scyatyke, sciatiche, syaticke, sciatique, seatick, sciatick, ciatico, sciatico, and sciatic.* Sciatica inspired the naming of a plant, the sciatica cress, which was suggested as a treatment in a sixteenth-century botanical catalogue (Turner, 1562). Sciatica crippled senators in Shakespearian drama (*Timon of Athens,* 1607).

Sciatic pains were confused, in those days even more than now, with hip pains and other types of back and leg pains. In the eighteenth century, a famous Italian physician who made many other important contributions to medical knowledge, Domenico Cotugno (1736–1822), described the type of sciatica that is amenable to modern-day surgical treatment. The clarity and detail of his description has not been much surpassed. Cotugno, however, knew very little of the causes of sciatica. The knowledge of the relationship of many cases of sciatica to ruptured intervertebral discs awaited better knowledge of those discs. Most of all, it awaited someone to put together the knowledge about discs with the knowledge about sciatica. In terms of the pace of modern-day medical advancements, it was a long wait.

Vesalius, a Roman physician, scientist, and artist who is widely regarded as the father of human anatomy, described the intervertebral disc as early as the second century. Much later, in 1858, Hubert von Luschka, a German pathologist, studied the human spine in great detail. Among Luschka's discoveries were *Knorpelanswuche,* which he described as bean-sized, gelatinous, soft, grayish masses that had eroded through the ligament that runs across the vertebral bodies. These are the same observations that surgeons who operate on patients with ruptured discs make regularly in modern operating rooms. Luschka's findings were on autopsy specimens in the morgue. He probably knew nothing of sciatica, or at least didn't put the two together. That didn't happen for almost 75 more years.

During those 75 years, some crucial things happened. Sterile technique for the control of infection during operations, general anesthesia, and the discovery of x rays were the most important. Those things increased the accuracy of diagnosis and the safety of surgical treatments, making the performance of spinal surgery much more commonplace than it had been. Surgeons who were involved with diagnosis of patients' symptoms were able to make observations of their anatomy. That closed the gap between what had been observed clinically by those providing medical treatments and what had been observed anatomically by those studying tissues from autopsy.

Isolated case reports of proven disc ruptures were reported shortly after the turn of the century. It was even suggested that they could cause sciatica, but not much attention was given to the suggestion. Over the first three decades of the twentieth century, surgical experience with removal of cartilage tumors or loose bodies from the vertebral canal greatly increased. The correlation between these and Luschka's *Knorpelanswuches* and Cotugno's sciatica came in the 1930s.

In the early 1930s, Joseph Seaton Barr, an orthopedic surgeon, called to the attention of William Jason Mixter, a neurological surgeon, that the soft, gray, bean-sized masses that neurosurgeons had been removing seemed identical to what Georg Schmorl, their contemporary leader of German pathologists, was calling ruptured fragments from the intervertebral disc. Barr and Mixter went to work on it at Massachusetts General Hospital, where they practiced. In 1934, they published a report on 19 patients surgically treated for ruptured intervertebral discs. That paper ushered in what has come to be known among spinal surgeons as the era of the disc.

Nineteen good results aren't scientific proof when dealing with all of the variables inherent in such a study. There were things about this report, however, that led otherwise skeptical physicians to accept the validity of correlating surgical removal of ruptured discs with relief of patients' pains. One was that the whole concept fit elegantly into what was already well-documented scientific fact about the anatomy and pathology of the region.

The other reason why this correlation was so readily accepted was based on who said it, where, and for what purpose. Perhaps that should not enter into purely scientific reasoning, but credibility weighs highly among physicians. They must accept the best information available for the treatment of their patients when pure, hard, scientific data are not always available. Mixter and Barr were highly respected physicians on the faculty at Harvard. Their paper was published in the *New England Journal of Medicine*. Today, that journal is quoted with regularity in media reports of medical progress. It came to that status because of many years of rigorous editorial integrity. Then, as now, physicians tended to trust what they read there more than information they might obtain from many other sources.

The reports of critical, relatively disinterested surgeons that removal of ruptured intervertebral discs could relieve back and sciatic pain dramatically led to widespread clinical use of the method. The application was mostly by surgeons whose reputations and livelihoods depended on the success of their treatments and who were, consequently, not in a position to be as objectively critical as those who were in established academic practices. Of course, if the method had had no merit, those in private practice would have quickly abandoned it. Given that it had some merit, it was hard for them to put it to the hard tests of scientific study to determine precisely for whom it should and should not be applied.

Sciatica usually is accompanied by low back pain. Back pain, a much more common symptom than sciatica, is seldom associated with true sciatica, but it is often accompanied by varying types of leg and hip pain. The dramatic successes of sciatica relief for the few patients of pioneers like Mixter and Barr led to the hope that the answer finally had been found for the ubiquitous problem of back pain. That hope became a belief for thousands of surgeons and millions of patients over the ensuing decades. The era of the disc, the time of widespread belief that back pain is caused by disorders of the intervertebral discs and can be relieved by surgical procedures on those discs, flourished in the 1940s and 1950s and has a persisting, though modified, influence today.

The ideas that back and sciatic pain come when a portion of the nucleus ruptures through the anulus and that removal of that nucleus would relieve the pain were crystallized by Mixter and Barr. Those ideas and the technical aspects of the surgery have endured with relatively little modification. They simply have been refined. The biggest change over the years has been in the selection process that tells doctors and patients who would and who would not be helped by surgery.

At this stage in the consideration of the evolution of disc surgery, we must note the influence of the Scandinavians. The ingenuity of American practitioners combined techniques of descriptive clinical medicine they had inherited from Greek, Italian, French, and English physicians and the knowledge of spinal abnormalities provided by the work of generations of German pathologists. The method they devised was to be scrutinized, tested, and critiqued most effectively by Scandinavians.

Just as there were cultural elements that set the stage for innovative surgery by Americans, there are circumstances that have made Sweden and Norway ideal locations for critical analysis. The populations of those countries are geographically confined and stable, making it easy to follow the course of a group of patients over a long time. The medical care delivery system and the research systems in the universities make complex, long-term studies of patient treatment methods much easier there than in most countries. For many reasons, the record stands in the analysis of back pain and back operations. The most thoroughly detailed and critical studies and the most enlightening human experiments have come from Scandinavia.

In the late 1930s, at the Karolinska Institute in Sweden, Sten Friberg began to study this whole matter of sciatica and discs and lumbar operations. With characteristic Swedish thoroughness, Friberg published a 114-page article (actually, *Acta Chiurgica Scandinavica,* the Scandinavian surgeons' equivalent to the *New England Journal of Medicine,* issues such long articles as self-contained supplements). Very little can be said today about these problems that Friberg did not say in that work of 1941.

While Swedish researchers and volunteers have made some important contributions to understanding the basic functions of the low back, perhaps their most important contribution has been to talk sense to the rest of the world. The slow evolution of discovering who would and who would not be helped by disc surgery has been led, or at least best articulated, by Friberg's successors as Swedish master back doctors—first Carl Hirsch and currently Alf Nachemson.

There was such a great wave of enthusiasm for disc surgery in the era of the disc that the overuse and misuse of the technique almost obscured the benefits. Criticism of the treatment came almost full circle to the point where there was doubt about the effectiveness. Through all of this, no one had really subjected disc excision for sciatica to the scrutiny of well-controlled scientific analysis.

Appropriately, it was a Scandinavian who, in 1978, finally published a study that seemed to lay some of the critical questions about effectiveness to rest. Henrik Weber, a Norwegian neurologist, designed a very tightly controlled, prospective, detailed study which he pursued and published after years of observations. For the first time, spinal surgeons could offer proof of what they had known all along, that surgical removal of a herniated disc, when performed for proper indications, is effective treatment. In the best Scandinavian tradition, the paper covered 64 pages of the *Journal of Oslo City Hospital*. In 1983 Weber substantiated his earlier work with a review of his data covering a ten-year span.

There have been some efforts to make what has finally proven to be a good thing better. Innovations and ingenuity with surgical technique have brought a few changes, though the techniques described by a number of American surgeons in the 1930s and digested by Friberg's 1941 article have remained the standard.

There has been a relatively recent flirtation, mostly American, with variations on technique that are called microsurgery. Most surgeons don't regard the various kinds of microsurgery as very different from standard technique. Opinions vary about whether they may be better or worse than the standard.

One form of microsurgery is so named because a microscope is used during part of the procedure. The microscope provides a magnified view of the nerve and the disc. Whether this is helpful or not is a matter of debate. Some surgeons who use microscopes also believe that only a small part of the nucleus should be removed. This "less is better" philosophy remains controversial with strongly opinioned and well-qualified professionals on both sides of the issues.

Another technique of microsurgery mimics the much more popular arthroscopic knee surgery. Nucleus material is removed through a pencil-sized tube inserted into the disc. This is not, at this time, a widely accepted technique, and it has many critics. There are fears that the point of contact of the disc with the nerve cannot be approached safely through such an exposure.

Scientific documentation of the effectiveness or ineffectiveness of relatively minor variations from standard technique is probably a long way off. After all, we waited 44 years in this fast-paced century for the standard to be properly tested. Besides all the testing problems previously described, an additional event has diverted the attention of investigators from surgical modifications. That event is the advent of chemonucleolysis.

Chemonucleolysis

Chemonucleolysis, a word derived from the idea that the nucleus of the disc is chemically dissolved, refers to the removal of a portion of the disc by injection of an enzyme directly into the disc. The events that led to the discovery and proven usefulness of chemonucleolysis span a shorter time but are no less convoluted than those described for surgery.

In 1928, during the course of research on the poisons produced by certain toxic bacteria, a curious phenomenon was observed. If a tiny amount of the toxin was injected just under the skin of a laboratory animal, a small area of inflammation, like a bee sting, occurred. If, however, an additional tiny amount was given through the veins of the animal 18 hours later, a large area of skin around the first injection site died. The researcher was Gregory Shwartzman, and the phenomenon became known as the Shwartzman reaction.

The Shwartzman reaction piqued the interest of a young physician named Lewis Thomas. This interest launched his career in medical research and journalism. Thomas's research has produced important scientific insights. His writings about the directions of medical science continue to stimulate thousands of readers to explore the romance of medical research.

Much medical discovery is by serendipity—luck, chance, and coincidence. Each new truth has an unanticipatable legacy. Gregory Shwartzman had no idea that he had launched the career of medical research's most articulate spokesman. Lewis Thomas had no anticipation that his investigation of the Shwartzman reaction would set off the most profound and controversial innovation in the treatment of disc disorders since Mixter and Barr popularized surgical disc excision.

Thomas knew that blood vessels ruptured during the Shwartzman reaction. This led him to experiment with enzymes that might dissolve components of blood vessel walls. Among the drugs he tried was papain, an enzyme from the latex of papaya. Papain was not a new drug. It had been used in the early 1940s to facilitate the withdrawal of fluid from ganglion cysts.

Thomas's papain experiments were done on rabbits. He found that papain was not a very satisfactory drug for inducing the Shwartzman reaction, but he noticed a strange, unexpected occurrence. As he pushed the dosage of intravenous papain higher, he noticed that the rabbits' ears wilted and drooped like those of cocker spaniels.

Thomas examined the rabbits' wilted ears and found the cells of the cartilage and the fibers of collagen to be unharmed. He found the occurrence amusing but not of much value to the research he was doing when he first noticed it in 1947. In 1953, he turned his attention to the subject again. This time, he found that the wilting occurred because the papain dissolved the cartilage matrix. The matrix is the amorphous mass of protein and carbohydrate that fills the spaces between the cells and fibers the way air fills a room around all of its contents.

At about the same time that Thomas first noticed that papain gave his rabbits spaniel ears, Carl Hirsch, one of Sweden's master back surgeons, was working on discograms. He learned to introduce a hypodermic needle into the center of lumbar discs. By injecting a small amount of x-ray dye through the needle, he could obtain x-ray images of the shape of the nucleus of the disc.

By the mid-1950s, discograms were in common use. The technique was used for diagnosis, but the ability to place an injection needle accurately in the center of the disc introduced obvious treatment possibilities. Henry Feffer, a pioneer in the use of the discogram in the United States, began a long trial of injection of cortisone-like medications into discs.

In 1959, Lyman Smith, an orthopedic surgeon in Chicago, learned about Lewis Thomas's rabbits. He thought papain might be helpful in the treatment of cartilage cancers. He tried it on chondrosarcomas in mice, but it didn't work. He did find, however, that it dissolved the nucleus of the intervertebral discs of rabbits.

By 1961, Smith, working with enzyme chemists at a large pharmaceutical laboratory, had tried a number of enzymes and found that chymopapain, one of the papaya enzymes, held the most promise as a drug to use for dissolving human disc tissue. That conclusion was based upon determinations of effectiveness and low toxicity. The drug seemed to be highly specific, working only on the mucoprotein matrix of the nucleus and leaving neighboring tissues unharmed.

By 1963, an investigational new drug application was made, and Smith had injected the first human patient with chymopapain. The drug was available to several clinical investigators, orthopedic and neurological surgeons, who were acquainted with techniques for using it and who agreed to report on complications and results.

Ideally, there are four phases for the investigation of new drugs. The first phase is animal experimentation. Following that, a double blind study, in which neither the doctor nor the patient knows whether the true drug or an ineffective substitute is being used, is performed on a relatively small number of patients who are aware that they are participating in an experiment. There are legal and ethical concerns about double blind studies, but, when there are a large number of factors to evaluate, it is an essential part of the investigative process. Phase three is the use of the drug for a large number of patients under controlled circumstances with careful documentation of results. General release for use by the medical profession is phase four.

In the case of chymopapain, phase two and phase three occurred out of sequence. A large number of patients were injected and a great deal of enthusiasm was engendered by the testimonials of patients and doctors before the treatment was subjected to the more scientific scrutiny of the double blind study.

The reasons for skipping phase two were not just ones of haste or carelessness. To be valid, the study must be done on patients who are truly suffering. To subject half of those patients to a treatment designed to be ineffective is distasteful to investigators and patients alike.

Even though we say we have the proof of good studies that surgery is effective, we don't really have that kind of proof. To do a double blind study on surgical treatment would require the treating physician to refer the patients to a surgeon who does not communicate with them. The surgeon would do the entire operation exactly the same for all patients except that, for half, the surgeon would only scratch around the ruptured discs and leave them pressing against the nerves and then send the patients back to the original doctor without telling either the patient or the doctor which patients had and which had not had the discs removed. This hasn't been done. But the situation with chemonucleolysis was nearly the same, and finally such studies were done. One difference that made it more palatable was that the false treatments—the injection of ineffective substances into the discs—were not likely to be as harmful for those patients as false surgeries would be.

While the third phase of chymopapain investigation—large number of patients under controlled circumstances—was being conducted in the 1960s, another enzyme—collagenase—entered phase one (animal experimentation). This set off a competition between the two drugs not unlike the scientific and sometimes political race that occurred during development of the polio vaccine in the 1940s.

Opponents of the use of chymopapain claimed that some patients had suffered devastating complications as a result of receiving the drug and that animal experiments had shown the drug was harmful to tissues other than disc contents. Proponents defended the drug, saying it was not responsible for the complications reported. They inferred that some of the animal experiments had been done improperly. Personalities and emotions clouded over an issue that was unclear from the beginning.

One problem about which there was not much controversy was a worry about allergic reactions. Chymopapain does not occur naturally in the body, and some people are allergic to it. The percentage of allergic people is small, but sometimes the reactions are very severe. Because of fear of inducing allergy, the original investigators agreed that they would use the drug only once on each patient. To use it again later might increase the risk of allergy, so it was agreed to eliminate that risk.

In 1972, after injecting the drug 900 times and being convinced of its effectiveness and safety, Lyman Smith violated his own rules. He injected a famous baseball player whom he had injected previously. There was no apparent ill effect to the baseball player, but by then the controversy over how and why chymopapain was to be used was heated. Smith's privileges to use the drug he had developed were withdrawn.

In 1973, a committee of past presidents of the American Academy of Orthopedic Surgeons reviewed the results of 37 investigating doctors who had injected 9000 patients with chymopapain. They concluded that it was safe and effective and asked that the U.S. Food and Drug Administration release the drug for phase four, general use.

Also in 1973, Bernard Sussman, a neurosurgeon from Washington D.C., pleaded that the FDA withdraw chymopapain. He said it was neither safe nor effective and that collagenase was a superior drug. In 1974, Henry Feffer reported on 244 patients who had been given cortisone-derivative drugs into their discs. He said the results had been good in about half.

In March 1974, the Surgical Drugs Advisory Committee of the FDA recommended that the new drug application for chymopapain be approved and that it be released for use by medical specialists. That fall, the FDA leaked the intent to publish notice in the *Federal Register* of release of chymopapain to phase four, an event that would call for full and open comment about the drug over the next 60 days. In anticipation of release of the drug, 1600 physicians, mostly orthopedic surgeons, attended courses in six American cities to learn how to use the drug.

The emotions and the objective uncertainties about chymopapain peaked at the time of the anticipation of release in 1974. Congressional committee hearings and pleadings before the FDA resulted in delay of the release. The plan was to go back to what had been passed over—phase two, the double blind study.

Double blind studies were conducted in four American hospitals on 104 patients. By that time, 13,700 patients had already received the drug.

In July 1975, the investigators who performed the double blind study reported that they had been unable to prove that chymopapain was any more effective than the supposedly inert substances that were given, unknown to both patient and doctor, to half of the patients. The conclusions of the FDA were that, though the drug was reasonably safe and had been proven experimentally to have effect on the discs, it had not been proven to be clinically effective in treatment of ruptured discs in humans. They recommended that the drug no longer be used except in further double blind study. Phase three study was then stopped and phase two continued.

Proponents of release of the drug criticized the double blind studies. They said there were too few patients, that the technique of injection had not always been correct, that the evaluation process was not good enough, that the placebo drug that was used was not inert, that the results had been evaluated too hastily, and that the dosage of chymopapain had been too small.

While small double blind studies continued to be the only use of chymopapain in the United States, the drug was available for more general use in Europe and Canada. Toronto became the referral center for many American patients whose doctors wanted them to be treated with chymopapain. By 1980, one orthopedic surgeon in Toronto reported that about 70 percent of the 2000 patients he had injected with chymopapain had been successfully relieved of pain.

In 1979, the FDA approved a small, tightly controlled study on the use of purified collagenase injected into ruptured human intervertebral discs. The early results of this study—being done by an orthopedic surgeon in New Jersey and another in Bogotá, Colombia—have been encouraging. An application for approval for phase four status, commercial availability for collagenase, was filed in 1983.

By 1981, the results of double blind studies in the United States and in Australia supported the contention that chymopapain was clinically effective. Those studies and the long-term success of the Canadian use of the drug renewed pressure for general release in the United States. In 1983, the drug was released for use by qualified medical specialists in the United States. Courses, cosponsored by the American Academy of Orthopedic Surgeons and the American Association of Neurological Surgeons, were attended by thousands of surgeons. Chymopapain had finally entered phase four of testing in the United States.

That chymopapain dissolves a portion of the human disc, that it can be given with reasonable safety, and that it can be used to relieve suffering from ruptured discs has been proven by more scientific method than is applied to most medical treatments. Whether or not it is safer and more effective than surgery remains controversial. Whether drugs other than chymopapain can be used in the same way with more safety and better effect remains unknown.

Complications from chymopapain occur in about 3 percent of cases. About half of those are allergic reactions. Some of the allergic reactions are of the severe, anaphylactoid type. Deaths occur in less than one in 1000. Since guidelines for selecting allergic patients are unreliable, these deaths cause serious concern about the safety of this treatment. Serum and skin tests to select those who may be allergic hold promise and are available, but reliable data about false positive and false negative reactions to these tests are not available.

Dissolving the disc by injection has some theoretical advantage over surgery. It may leave less scar around the nerve than an operation does. Less scar may mean a better result for some people.

Some patients don't get better after chemonucleolysis. If the reason is that a piece of ruptured disc is not reached by the injected enzyme, subsequent operation to remove that disc fragment may still give a good result.

Hopes for the future include the discovery of drugs for injection that are safer and more effective than chymopapain, better ability to distinguish allergy and other risk factors for specific patients, and better means of predicting which patients would be treated most effectively by surgery and which by injection. Those hopes depend upon new discoveries. They also depend upon the experience gained from phase four use of chymopapain and the comparisons that will be drawn between it and other treatments.

Nonscientific Treatments

No treatments for back pain have endured the scrutiny that has been applied to surgery and to chemonucleolysis. That includes most of the recommendations for treatment made in this book. The bases for those recommendations have been that they have been found to have some success from a large experience and that they make sense.

The use of medicine for back pain usually is offered with full awareness on the part of both patient and physician that the purpose is to ease symptoms. There is no expectation that the medicine really is a cure. Testing of these medicines is, therefore, designed to evaluate the effect on a specific symptom, such as pain or anxiety, rather than on the underlying condition. Most prescription medicines have been tested adequately for safety and effectiveness in relief of the symptoms for which they are intended. Some medications have not been tested in that way or have failed those tests. Some medications are used for symptoms for which they have not been tested appropriately. Those problems are discussed in Chapter 6.

There are variations of physical therapy that are offered as symptom relieving, even curative treatments for back disorders. Gravity traction is one of contemporary interest, as discussed in Chapter 1. Acupuncture is another. The safer and easier analogue—acupressure—has been considered here. Claims for therapeutic effect of acupuncture beyond transient pain relief and muscle relaxation have not been substantiated by trials done by scientific methods. Perhaps it is unfair to subject this ancient oriental healing technique to the standards of western science.

Manipulation is an ancient treatment method that must be taken seriously because its proponents have endured and transcended centuries, cultures, and educational biases. There have been serious and worthy attempts to provide scientific documentation of the clinical effectiveness of manipulation, and, though some results have been positive, the best available data lead to conflicting conclusions.

One of the great problems with trying to critique manipulation is that it has been used for such a great variety of problems, by such a great variety of practitioners, with such a wide range of expectations. Friar Moulton, an Augustinian monk, authored *The Compleat Bonesetter* in the seventeenth century. This was basically a treatise on manipulation treatments for various skeletal disorders. Manipulation had been a part of medical practice from classical times in Europe and continues to be today.

One of the problems with accepting manipulation as a scientifically valid treatment is that we don't know what it really does on the level of basic anatomy and physiology. Theories have been advanced that spinal manipulation may shift a misplaced nucleus to a better place in the disc, that it can pop a trapped piece of joint lining out of a facet joint, that it can release a facet joint that is hung on a little bony ridge on the facet, that it can free a tiny nerve twig from within a facet joint, or that it can break loose scar adhesions around a disc or a facet joint. While all of these things are theoretically possible, it is very hard for those who regularly look at the anatomy of the living human back in the operating room to believe that any of those things occur very often and especially that they could occur on any predictable basis as a result of manipulation.

Other explanations for the positive effects of manipulation are that it may break up reflex arcs of pain, spasm, and stiffness, and that it has a very reassuring psychological effect. Such functional explanations for the undeniable fact that manipulation has helped a lot of people are easier for surgeons to accept than are mechanical explanations based on the theories mentioned above. The observation of so-called minor vertebral derangements on x rays are regarded by most physicians either as variations of normal, like big feet or crooked noses, or as normal changes of aging, like skin wrinkles.

Many physicians recognize the benefits—scientific or not—of manipulation. This is true more in Europe than in the United States. Many American physicians may be reactionary in their criticism of the method because of what they have perceived to be abuses. Most of the benefits can be derived, and the abuses avoided, by learning self-care techniques of first aid and exercise.

Being a Patient

Back pain usually can be prevented and self-treated without the help of professionals. But there are exceptions. You could need professional help for diagnosis so you can be sure the problem is something you can manage yourself. Some aspect of your problem could require specialized treatment measures beyond what you can self-administer. You should select the type of professional help according to your particular need.

How to Choose a Professional. Basic identifying characteristics of professionals are their academic degrees. The fact that someone is called "Doctor" tells you nothing about skills or qualifications—he or she could be a professional basketball player. Not all professionals who call themselves physicians are medical doctors.

The letters that follow the name identify the academic qualification. M.D. means medical doctor and indicates that the professional has graduated from medical school. M.D. does not necessarily mean licensed to practice medicine. Licensure is a function of government regulation and requires good standing in addition to an appropriate degree.

Osteopaths possess the D.O. degree. Osteopaths graduate from a school of osteopathy rather than from a medical school. Licensing requirements for D.O.s and M.D.s are very similar. Osteopathy was founded in 1874 by Andrew Taylor Still, an American country doctor. Osteopathy originally relied upon spinal malalignment as an explanation for human disease and upon manipulation as treatment. Osteopathy evolved to embrace the principles and teachings of traditional medicine. Though some osteopaths still use spinal manipulation in much of their practices, most of the approximately 20,000 D.O.s in the U.S. practice medicine along the same lines as do M.D.s. Doctors of osteopathy may specialize, as do medical doctors. Most hospitals accord privileges to D.O.s as they do to M.D.s.

The degree of Ph.D., doctor of philosophy, is the highest academic degree awarded in most fields of learning. Some Ph.D.s work in health-related fields and may offer professional services to patients. Psychologists are the Ph.D.s who are most likely to diagnose or treat some back pain problems.

Physical therapists must be registered to practice and designate themselves as R.P.T., registered physical therapist. To be eligible for registration, physical therapists now must be graduates from either a four year university program or a two year postgraduate program. Physical therapists are expert at administration of passive treatment modalities such as heat, ice, massage, ultrasound, and mobilization. They teach exercise, body mechanics, relaxation, and other active self-care techniques. Some physical therapists specialize in back care and may direct back schools. They are trained in physical diagnosis but are limited in the diagnostic methods they may employ. In most American states physical therapists may treat only by medical prescription.

Chiropractors have the degree D.Ch. They are called doctors and physicians but are not graduates of medical or osteopathic schools. They are graduates of schools of chiropractic. Chiropractic was founded in 1895 by D.D. Palmer, an Iowa grocer, who claimed to cure deafness by spinal manipulation. The philosophical approach to diagnosis and treatment by chiropractic is quite different from that of medicine. The basic premise of chiropractic is that pain and disease results from spinal malalignment; that if you have symptoms, your spine is malaligned and you need chiropractic treatment. Examinations and x rays only confirm and localize what is a foregone conclusion. Some chiropractors confine their practices to musculoskeletal disorders and their treatments to conventional physical therapeutic methods and nutritional counselling, while others adhere to the traditional chiropractic doctrines that spinal manipulation is appropriate treatment for a wide range of diseases.

Many chiropractors are skilled and compassionate people who have relieved the suffering of many patients. The objection most medical doctors have to the way most chiropractors practice is that chiropractors designate variations of normal anatomy as sources of disease. Based on those diagnoses, they treat people who should have more definitive diagnostic testing or, most often, who should simply be reassured and encouraged in self-care methods. Of course, not all chiropractors are guilty and not all medical doctors are blameless of such practices.

Among medical doctors, there are many specialists who may help with the diagnosis or treatment of back pain. If you don't know where to turn, it is best to start with your family doctor or internal medicine specialist. Your family doctor may be able to provide the service you need and, if not, could direct you to the most appropriate specialist.

The specialists who examine most people for the biggest variety of back pain problems are orthopedic surgeons. Though orthopedists are surgical specialists, most of them spend about half their professional lives providing diagnostic and nonsurgical care. Some orthopedic surgeons subspecialize in back care or spinal surgery.

Neurosurgeons perform lumbar disc surgery and chemonucleolysis in basically the same way as orthopedists. Differences in styles and techniques are greater among individuals than between the two surgical disciplines.

The nonsurgeon medical doctors who provide specialty care for low back pain are neurologists, physiatrists, rheumatologists, industrial medicine physicians, psychiatrists, anesthesiologists, and radiologists. Neurologists specialize in diagnosis and nonsurgical treatment of diseases of the nervous system. Physiatrists are rehabilitation specialists who treat patients with chronic pain and disability. Rheumatologists are medical doctors who specialize in the diagnosis and treatment of arthritis. Rheumatologists usually care for back pain problems when the diagnosis is uncertain or when long-term management of arthritis medications is needed. Industrial physicians often become specialists in back care because back pain is such a common complaint among workers. Psychiatrists care for back pain if psychotherapy, long-term medication for anxiety or depression, or medication withdrawal are needed. Anesthesiologists perform diagnostic nerve blocks and inject therapeutic medicines into the spinal canal. Radiologists do x-ray diagnosis testing.

Some back pain problems are evaluated and treated by a combination of professionals or a clinic. An established combination of specialists routinely may examine back pain patients at some large referral centers. They make a consensus diagnosis and treatment recommendation.

Pain clinics, also called pain control centers or pain management units, are multispecialty endeavors that treat complex chronic pain problems. Most pain clinic teams include a physician, a psychologist, a social worker, and a physical therapist. They may include a rehabilitation specialist who coordinates the efforts of the rest of the team with an effort at vocational readjustment. The physician is usually a physiatrist, neurologist, orthopedic surgeon, or anesthesiologist. Those in the other specialties mentioned above are at least available for consultation. Treatment programs usually include drug withdrawal, behavior modification, nerve blocks, and self-care methods.

Back schools emphasize self-care measures. Most are administered by physical therapists. Physician specialists advise and sometimes participate. Back schools add the dimension of direct personal teaching to the treatment and prevention philosophies espoused in this book.

How to be a Patient. Regardless of the circumstances of your need or the professional you choose, there are some things that will make you a better patient. Being a good patient does not mean being a patient who is no trouble; it means being a patient who makes an honest effort to help guide the doctor toward an accurate diagnosis and successful treatment.

You need to tell the doctor why you are there and what you expect. Many people play "you are the doctor, you tell me what is wrong" games with their doctors. Accurate medical diagnosis is difficult enough when all of the concerns and facts are known. The doctor needs the important facts and needs to know what worries you have about your health.

If you are worried about cancer, you need to tell that to the doctor. If you have a change in bowel habits or painful urination or problems with sexual performance, tell it to the doctor. If you are worried about x rays and don't want them done, let your concern be known. If you are worried that too many or too few tests will be done, tell the doctor about it. If you have been to other doctors or have had other opinions or treatments, don't keep it a secret. If your major concern is to obtain a medical opinion for insurance, a lawsuit, or social security, tell the doctor that.

Competent, experienced doctors have a keen sense of what is true and what isn't about medical symptoms. They have an accurate feel for what are and what are not valid responses to an examination. Even if you are frustrated by earlier experiences or worried that the doctor will not be sufficiently impressed, don't exaggerate your symptoms and responses. Attempts to falsify or exaggerate medical findings only make the situation more difficult for you and could endanger your health.

Don't be modest about your body during a medical examination. Rectal or pelvic examinations are sometimes done as part of an evaluation for back pain. If you have concern about either, don't be afraid to ask. If you wish for a nurse to be present during the examination, request it.

Some doctors permit friends and relatives to be present during an examination and some do not. If you would rather not have them present and are reluctant to ask them to leave, ask the doctor or the nurse to excuse them for you. If you wish a relative to be present and the doctor permits it, don't allow the relative to interfere with the examination. Unless the doctor specifically addresses a question to the relative, the questions are meant for your response alone.

When the tests and recommendations are complete, you should tell the doctor what you think. If you think there should be more tests or different treatments, say so. The doctor may not agree, but it is best for what you are thinking to be known.

If you wish another opinion, request it. Many people shop around for doctors and don't ever tell any one doctor what they are really looking for, where else they have been, or what else they have been told. Doctors have different styles of explaining things, and unless you let each doctor know what you are worried about, what else has been done, and what you have been told, you may endure a lot of needless, expensive, and sometimes harmful repetition of tests and treatments.

Professional Examinations. Examinations by a doctor usually begin with a history, a question-and-answer session about the problem. The history may be preceded by a written questionnaire or an interview with a nurse, but don't be afraid to repeat what you think is important or to add facts when you are examined by the doctor.

The history is followed by a physical examination. The type and detail of the examination will vary according to the needs suggested by the history. There are several tests that may add important information to the history and physical findings.

Blood and Urine Tests. A blood count, a battery of serum tests, and a urinalysis may be needed for general health screening. Such an approach to back pain is more likely to be taken by your family doctor or an internist. Such testing is especially appropriate if your symptoms include loss of energy, weight loss, fever, weakness, or other symptoms not directly related to your lower back.

Blood tests for various forms of arthritis may be done if your symptoms suggest the need for them. X-ray findings sometimes raise questions about arthritis, tumors, or bone diseases, which are best answered by information provided by blood tests.

X Ray. Most specialists who examine you for persistent low back pain will request that you have x rays taken of your lumbar spine. Three pictures are standard. Occasionally, more are needed to examine your hips and upper back or to look at the lumbar area from oblique angles or in different positions.

Each x ray of this type subjects you to a small dose of radiation. Too much radiation can be harmful. Unfortunately, there are no reliable ways to know exactly how much is too much, what the harmful effects will be, or when they will be manifest. Some body areas are more vulnerable to radiation. In the case of low back x rays in young people, the major concern is about the reproductive organs.

You are exposed to a normal amount of radiation from sunlight and earth minerals. The amount of radiation from one low back x ray is about the same as from a year of normal exposure.

Roentgen discovered the x ray just before the turn of the century. Since then, x rays have been used a great deal for medical diagnosis. Based upon this huge experience, it seems very unlikely that harm results from the doses of x ray used for most diagnoses. It is clear, however, that large doses of x ray are harmful. Since we don't know for certain about small doses and since some individuals may be particularly vulnerable, it is best to avoid unnecessary x rays.

You want x rays to help diagnose your back pain if the benefits to be gained outweigh the risks. Pregnant women and people who have had large x-ray exposures in the past are at increased risk. Young people should be more cautious about having x rays than older people.

Benefits of x ray depend upon your worries and the doctor's uncertainty about diagnosis. Doctors can predict with a high degree of accuracy whether or not the x ray is going to reveal anything important. That is not 100 percent so, but if you are worried about cancer or something else seriously wrong with your bones, the x ray may be worthwhile for the added reassurance. If there are important social issues at stake, the information provided by x ray to help settle them may be worth the risk.

If you weigh the risks and benefits and think you might rather not have an x ray, talk to the doctor about it. If the doctor is reasonably certain the x ray won't show anything important and you are willing to accept the risk of missing something that may have been revealed by x ray, then the two of you may choose to defer an x-ray examination.

CAT Scans. Computerized axial tomography (CAT, sometimes just CT) is a modification of x-ray examination made possible by the marriage of an x-ray machine and a computer. X rays are done at multiple angles, and the information is fed into a computer. Once the data are in the computer, images of the subject can be constructed in various planes without additional radiation. Unlike conventional x ray, CAT scanning may produce a cross-section picture. The doctor can look right into the vertebral canal instead of just seeing through it from front and side.

CAT scans are more expensive, and the radiation dose is higher than regular x rays. The radiation dosage is more equivalent to contrast x-ray studies such as myelograms. CAT scans of the lumbar spine do not require injection of a dye, an advantage over myelograms.

Experience with CAT scans has been brief. Many surgeons who have come to trust the information they obtain from myelograms have been unwilling to make surgical decisions based upon CAT scan findings.

Myelograms. Contrast material (dye) may be injected safely into the spinal fluid either in the lumbar area or at the base of the skull. Either water-soluble or oil-base contrast can be used. In most cases, water-soluble contrast injected into the lumbar area is used for low back pain diagnosis.

As with all drugs, there are some risks to being injected with myelogram dye. Serious allergic reactions and locally severe inflammatory reactions that produce scars around the spinal nerves have occurred. Such reactions are quite rare.

Many people have a fear of myelograms that is out of proportion to the risks. The discomfort and the risks are certainly more than you want to endure unnecessarily. If you need the examination, however, you should be reassured that, for the great majority of people, it is a safe and well-tolerated procedure.

The flow of x-ray dye may be observed by the radiologist using fluoroscopy. Individual x-ray exposures are made of the areas of interest. Radiation exposure varies with the amount of fluoroscopy and the number of exposures. Total exposure is within what are considered safe diagnostic limits under most circumstances.

Bone Scans. The advent of CAT scans and NMR scans has created confusion over what is meant by a bone scan. Bone scan is the commonly used term for scintimetry, the technique of creating an image by mapping the locations of radioactive isotopes in bone.

A tiny dose of radioactive mineral is injected into a vein. After enough time for the mineral to have been incorporated into the bone crystals, the radioactivity of the bones is mapped.

Bone scans are very sensitive but not very specific. Anything that causes increased formation of bone crystals will produce a hot spot on the bone scan. Abnormalities too small to be seen on regular x rays sometimes will appear on bone scans. Bone scans sometimes can be too sensitive, appearing abnormal where no important abnormality exists.

Like many x-ray examinations, radiation exposure from bone scans is not excessive but should not be ignored. Otherwise, bone scans are harmless and painless.

Ultrasound. Ultrasound is used to discover abnormal masses in much the same way as sonar is used by ships at sea. The sound rays are harmless.

There is no radiation exposure. The technique has not been satisfactory for use in the spine but may help in the search for unusual causes of back pain such as aneurysms of the aorta and tumors within the abdomen and pelvis.

NMR Scans. Nuclear magnetic resonance (NMR) has been used by chemists to determine the composition of samples since the 1930s. In England in the 1970s, adaptations of technique led to the use of NMR on humans. By the mid-1980s, it will be in widespread use on patients. NMR may replace many current examinations that require x ray.

To be examined by NMR, you are placed in a strong magnetic field, which seems to be harmless since many people have worked under such conditions without apparent ill effect. Subatomic particles align themselves in response to the magnet. Harmless radio waves are passed through your body. Radio signals received in response to the interaction between the radio waves and the aligned particles are computer analyzed. The computer can construct an image in any plane.

NMR has the potential for greater precision in some examinations than any available x-ray techniques. It does not require injection of dye and is probably harmless. The promise of NMR is great, but the experience is very brief. The risks, limitations, and capabilities of this innovation will be much better known after a few years of use.

Thermography. Abnormal nerve function may produce changes in skin temperature in the distribution of the nerve. Maps of skin surface temperature, called thermograms, may depict such changes. Experience with this test has been brief. It is harmless but somewhat time-consuming and expensive. Variations from normal on thermograms cannot be assumed to be caused by specific anatomic abnormalities, nor can they be assumed to correlate with pain.

EMG. Electromyography (EMG) and nerve conduction velocities (NCV) are tests that amplify the electrical activity of nerves and muscles. EMG is similar to electrocardiography (EKG), the tracing of heart muscle electricity. For EMG, insulated pins are inserted through the skin into individual muscles. Electrical activity from an electrode on the skin or in nearby tissue is subtracted from the activity at the pin tip; the difference is amplified and displayed on a cathode ray screen. Because movements of the muscle and the pin change the activity on the screen, EMG—unlike EKG—must be interpreted as it is performed. EMGs are performed by neurologists, physiatrists, and some orthopedists and neurosurgeons. EMGs are safe and minimally painful.

NCV is a measurement of the speed at which a shock travels along a nerve. It is done on the same machine as an EMG and often along with the EMG. The shock is mild and harmless except to anyone who must avoid shocks because of a cardiac pacemaker.

Interpretation of EMGs done for low back conditions can be difficult. Minor abnormalities may occur for a variety of reasons. Sometimes the nerve abnormalities are obvious without the need for electrical testing. Under certain circumstances, though, the information from EMG and NCV tests can be very important.

16
BEYOND READING
THIS BOOK

Some things you learn in this book are interesting but may not apply to your problem. Some apply during this learning process and then diminish in importance. Some apply when your back hurts and not when it doesn't—they can be tucked away to be pulled out in time of need. Others are of continuing and lasting importance.

Sometimes you too easily let what you have learned slip away, only to slide back into old habits. The challenge now is to find what is in your life to make the important changes permanent.

Very few people have the discipline and the drive to maintain difficult changes all alone. Of course, the responsibility and the main energy must come from you. One of the best ways to make sure you have fulfilled your obligations to yourself is to involve other people. They can't do it for you, but they can encourage you. Their help can keep you going through hard times if you know that failing would be failing them as well as yourself.

Your spouse, your family, and those closest to you need to know about your struggle and be involved in all phases of it. Having more casual friends, acquaintances, and coworkers know what you are doing also helps. Boring them with accounts of your symptoms and your difficulties doesn't help you or them, but hearing about your successes inspires them. Everyone is involved in personal struggles and takes inspiration from the success of others. Sharing your successes commits you to maintaining them. If you get lazy and slack off on your commitment, you risk disappointing others and yourself.

One particularly good way to combine social and personal commitments is to join new group activities that complement your efforts. Athletic associations, swim clubs, track clubs, health spas, and dance groups offer exercise programs that combine enjoyable forms of exercise with the stimulation and encouragement of group membership. Church, medical, and other encounter groups, discussion groups, or group therapy sessions provide the same thing for the psychosocial aspects of the problem. Workers' organizations, business organizations, or labor management forums may provide places to discuss relationships between back pain and work.

Beyond yourself, your family, your friends, and your community, things that are wrong with the whole culture make it difficult to resolve the problems created by back pain. Careers need to be designed for a lifetime so that adjustments are made in the demands of work for those who can no longer do what they once could. Unions and management need to recognize and push for working conditions that prevent excessive back strain. Workers need exercise breaks more than coffee breaks. Most people need exercise at noon a lot more than they need lunch. Recreation must mean personal involvement and satisfaction and not just watching a few superstars exercise on television. A pervasive attitude exists that health problems are someone else's responsibility—the doctor, the employer, the government, the family. Those attitudes must change, and society must pressure people to be well rather than encourage them to be sick.

This culture is full of people who don't exercise enough, who are overweight, who do jobs that are poorly designed, who are ignorant about how to accomplish work efficiently and safely, who don't know how to do anything about it and are afraid to try. The solution has to be education that is understood and practiced. Doing things right yourself is the first step toward reaching that solution. When you have finished this book, you will already be ahead of most people. Keep right on going, and get all that is in it for you. As you do, teach some others and push for changes that will make it better for everyone.

GLOSSARY

Abdomen: Portion of the trunk below the chest, above the pelvis, and in front of the spine.

Abdominal Muscles: Muscles that support and form the walls of the abdominal cavity; extend from the ribs to the pelvis and lumbar spine.

Abduction: Pulling away from the center of the body as in spreading the legs apart.

Abductors: Muscles from the pelvis to the femur (thigh bone) along the side of the hip.

Achilles Tendon: Tendon of the calf muscles; attaches to the heel. *Also called* Heel cord.

Active Exercise: Exercise done by using the force of one's own muscles with no outside assistance.

Acupressure: Technique of pressing against certain points on the body in an effort to relieve pain.

Acupuncture: Technique of placing pins into certain points on the body in an effort to relieve pain.

Adduction: Pulling toward the center of the body as in pulling the legs in to squeeze the knees together.

Adductors: Muscles from the pelvis to the inside border of the femur (thigh bone).

Adjustment: With reference to the spine, usually means an attempt to correct some malalignment or loss of motion by manipulation.

Adversarial: Refers to method of settling legal disputes in which the involved parties present opposing viewpoints.

Aerobic Dancing: Rhythmic exercise usually done to music; continuous action with no rest periods but not leading to breathlessness.

Analgesic: Medicine for the relief of pain.

Anaphylaxis (Anaphylactoid): Severe allergic reaction involving shock.

Anatomy: Study of the form of the body.

Anesthesiologist: Medical doctor who specializes in administration of medication to control pain.

Aneurysm: Abnormal enlargement of part of a blood vessel, usually of a large artery.

Ankylosing Spondylitis: Particular arthritic disease that affects the spine. *Also called* Marie-Strumpell's disease *or* Rheumatoid spondylitis.

Anterior: Toward the front, as opposed to *posterior,* which means toward the back.

Anthropormorphics: Measurements of standard human dimensions usually for the purpose of designing clothing or furniture.

Antidepressant: Medicine for the relief of feelings of depression.

Anti-inflammatory: Any drug or other agent (ice, for example) used to control inflammation.

Anulus Fibrosus: Ring-shaped ligament that attaches above and below to vertebral bodies and surrounds the nucleus pulposus of the intervertebral disc.

Arthritis: Disorder manifested by inflammation of joints; sometimes used imprecisely to mean anything that causes pain around joints.

Atherosclerosis: Change in arteries manifested by deposits of placques along the inside walls of the arteries.

Back School: Back treatment facility that emphasizes self-care and preventive measures.

Ballistic Exercise: Rapidly repeating, bouncing exercise efforts.

Biofeedback: Teaching relaxation and pain control by using devices that make one more aware of the body's tensions.

Body of a Vertebra: Block-shaped portion of the vertebra, located at the front of the spine. *Also called* Centrum.

Bone Scan: Mapping of bone activity using an injected radioisotope. *Also called* Scintimetry.

Bone Spur: See Osteophyte.

Bursa: Filmy, moist lubricating sac, usually located over joints and bony prominences.

Bursitis: Inflammation of a bursa; sometimes used imprecisely to mean any painful condition of the tissues around a joint.

Calcium Deposit: Calcium crystals in tissues other than bones, usually a response to injury or inflammation.

Calisthenics: Exercises done in series, usually in rhythm.

Cancer: Disease manifested by the growth of cells that are destructive to normal tissue and have the potential to spread to other areas.

Cardio-pulmonary Resuscitation: Technique of reviving a person who has stopped breathing or whose heart has stopped beating.

Cartilage: Body tissue commonly located at the ends of long bones; provides gliding surface and cushion for joints.

CAT Scan: Computerized axial tomography; computer-assisted x-ray technique of providing images in various planes. *Also called* CT scan.

Center of Gravity: Center of body weight; the axis about which a suspended body would rotate.

Centrum: See Body of a vertebra.

Cerebrospinal Fluid (CSF): Watery fluid that bathes the brain and spinal cord within the space contained by the meninges.

Cervical: Referring to the neck.

Chemonucleolysis: Technique of dissolving disc contents by injecting a chemical into the disc.

Chiropractic: Discipline based on the theory that many symptoms and disorders are explained by spinal malalignment.

Chondral Plate: Bone along the top and bottom surfaces of the body of each vertebra. *Also called* End plate.

Chymopapain: Enzyme, derived from papaya, used to dissolve disc contents.

Coccydynia: Pain in the coccyx.

Coccyx: Tail bone; four or five small vertebrae at the tip of the spine.

Collagen: Protein that is a major component of scars, ligaments, tendons, and the nonmineral portion of bone.

Collagenase: Enzyme that breaks down collagen; sometimes used for chemonucleolysis.

Compression Fracture: Crushing of the body of a vertebra.

Connective Tissues: Body tissues that bind one body part to another and fill the spaces between body parts.

Contour Position: Body position with hips and knees flexed and back supported.

Contrast Material: Material injected to fill spaces so the spaces will show clearly on x rays. *Also called* Dye.

Contrast Relaxation Exercise: Exercise to produce relaxation by experiencing first tension and then relaxation of certain muscles.

Cortex: Outer shell of bone; hard, compact portion of bone.

Corticosteroid: Any of the group of cortisone-like hormones or derived drugs. *Also called* Steroid.

Cortisone: Hormone formed by the adrenal gland. Chemically derived drugs, often used for their effect of reducing inflammation, may be called cortisone, corticosteroids, or steroids.

CSF: See Cerebrospinal fluid.

CT Scan: See CAT scan.

Cumulative Trauma: Injury that results from the added effects of repeated minor injuries.

Curvature: Variation from straight; with reference to the spine, sometimes used to mean scoliosis.

Defendant: Accused party in a legal action.

Degeneration: Changes of aging or changes similar to those that occur naturally with aging.

Diagonals: With reference to body mechanics, technique of positioning the body during stressful activities so that forces are taken through the body from one arm to the opposite leg.

Disability: Inability to function, usually because of some physical or emotional handicap.

Disc: Intervertebral disc; joints between the vertebral bodies; composed of a circular ligament, the anulus fibrosus, and a gel-like center, the nucleus pulposus. *Sometimes spelled* Disk.

Disc Degeneration: Loss of volume and water content of the nucleus of a disc, often accompanied by bone spurs at the attachments of the surrounding ligaments.

Disc Space: Space between the end plate of one vertebral body and that of the adjacent vertebral body.

Discectomy: Surgical removal of a portion of an intervertebral disc.

Discogram: X-ray study of a disc done after injection of contrast material into the disc.

Disk: See Disc.

Displacement Activity: Action performed as a substitute for one that is forbidden.

Dorsal: Thoracic or chest portion of the spine; also may designate direction, in which case it means nearly the same as posterior or toward the back.

Double Blind Study: Method of investigation in which neither the subject nor the investigator knows if the agent being tested is actually being used.

Dowager's Hump: Hunchback posture of the upper dorsal spine, common in older women with osteoporosis.

Dye: See Contrast material.

Dysfunction: Abnormal or irregular function or absence of normal function.

Elastic Abdominal Binder: Extensible band that may be pulled around the body to support the abdomen and lower back.

Electromyography (EMG): Recording and analysis of electrical activity in muscle.

EMG: See Electromyography.

End Plate: Chondral plate.

Endometriosis: Disorder of female reproductive organs manifested by abnormal occurrence of cells like those that line the uterus.

Endorphins: Naturally occurring hormones that reduce sensitivity to pain.

Enthesis: Site where tendons and ligaments bind to bone.

Ergonomics: Study of the accomplishment of work.

Extended: Brought to a straight line; opposite of *flexed*.

Extension: Stretched out straight; sometimes may mean beyond straight when used to mean the opposite of *flexion* (for example, bending the lower back to look up to the ceiling is extension of the back).

Facet: Bony processes on the posterior side of each vertebra.

Facet Joints: Joints where adjacent vertebrae articulate at the back of the spine.

Femur: Thigh bone.

Fibroid Tumors: Benign tumors of the uterus.

Fibrosis: Increase in the fiber content of a tissue; scarred.

Fibrositis Syndrome: Combination of multiple tender areas in muscles, fatigue, and sleep disorder; not associated with any known disease.

Fibrous: Composed of fibers; rope-like.

Flexed: Bent; opposite of *extended.*

Flexibility: Movability; freedom of motion of joints and muscles.

Flexion: Motion toward a bent position; opposite of *extension.*

Foramen (Foramina, plural): Hole or window, usually through or between bones.

Foraminal Stenosis: Narrowing of a foramen; with reference to the back, means narrowing of the intervertebral foramen.

Fusion: Surgical operation to eliminate motion.

Genitourinary Organ: Organs of sex and urine excretion.

Glycoproteins: Molecules composed of protein and carbohydrates, present in cartilage and nucleus pulposus.

Gravity Traction: Gravity-assisted pull on the body, such as by hanging upside-down or suspending oneself by crutches.

Greater Trochanter: Bony knob at the outer, upper side of the thigh bone.

Guided Imagery: Formation and manipulation of visual images of pain or other abstract problems.

Habituated: Having a strong desire for something though not an absolute physical need for it.

Hamstrings: Muscles of the back of the thigh.

Heel Cord: See Achilles tendon.

Hemilaminectomy: Operation done by removing the lamina from one side of one vertebra.

HLA–B27 Antigen: Blood test for a genetic configuration that has statistical implications about the presence of certain forms of arthritis.

Holistic: Embracing the whole experience of an individual as opposed to concentrating on some particular aspect.

Hormones: Naturally occurring chemicals produced by the body to regulate various body functions.

Ice Massage: Movement of ice over an area of soreness or tightness.

Iliac Arteries: Large arteries of the pelvis that derive from the aorta.

Iliotibial Band: Large muscle–tendon from the pelvis, along the outside of the thigh, to below the knee.

Ilium: Largest bone of the pelvis; bone felt at the waist.

Impairment: Physical limitation of function, independent of skills or motivation.

Inflammation: Reaction of the body to some irritating stimulus; characterized by swelling, redness, local increase in temperature, and tenderness.

Intervertebral Disc: Joints of the front of the spine, between adjacent vertebral bodies; composed of anulus fibrosus and nucleus pulposus.

Intervertebral Foramen: Window between the sides of adjacent vertebrae.

Ischial Tuberosities: Bony knobs at bottom of pelvic bone; pressure points when sitting upright.

Joints: Sites where adjacent bones make contact.

Kyphosis: Backward pointing curve of the spine; in the dorsal spine, up to about 45 degrees of kyphosis is normal.

Lamina: Portion of the vertebra that makes the back roof over the vertebral canal from each side of the midline spinous process to the side wall pedicles.

Laminectomy: Operation done by removal of the lamina; often loosely used to refer to any operation in which the vertebral canal is approached from the back side.

Lateral: To the side or from the side, as opposed to *medial*.

Lateral Recess: Space in the anterior corners of the vertebral canal, under the medial edge of the facets.

Ligament: Supporting structure from one bone to another; composed of fibers.

Ligamentum Flavum: Ligaments between adjacent laminae; very elastic and with a yellow color. *Also called* Yellow ligament.

List: Leaning of the body to one side so that the shoulders are not squarely above the hips.

Litigant: Individual involved in a lawsuit.

Little League Parent Syndrome: Backache caused by prolonged sitting on bleachers.

Lordosis: Forward-pointing curvature of the spine; some lordosis is normal in the lumbar and cervical spines.

Lumbar: Region of the back between the lowest ribs and the pelvis.

Lupus: Common short name used for systemic lupus erythematosis, a disease of unknown origin which affects multiple organs. Lupus also sometimes may refer to a skin disease.

Manipulation: Bending, twisting, or stretching action in attempt to produce a favorable change in the position or movement of muscles, joints, or bones.

Marie-Strumpell's Disease: See Ankylosing spondylitis.

Matrix: The space between; the fill space in which more-defined objects are located; like the air in a room.

Mechanical back pain: Back pain that occurs because the supporting structures of the back are not able to withstand the forces applied to them.

Medial: Toward the midline, as opposed to *lateral*.

Meditation: Relaxation through attention to breathing or other solitary diversion from ordinary concerns.

Meningeal Sac: Container formed by the meninges; holds cerebrospinal fluid.

Meninges: Thin tissue coverings that encase the spinal cord and brain and the fluid that bathes them.

Menopause: In women, time of changes in hormone function that occurs in middle life; signaled by cessation of menstruation.

Motor Point: Site where nerve joins muscle; frequently pain-sensitive.

Mucopolysaccharides: Complex carbohydrate molecules that have the capacity to hold water; present in the nucleus pulposus.

Muscle Relaxants: Medicines meant to relieve the pain that accompanies muscle tension.

Myelogram: X-ray study in which a contrast material is injected into the spinal fluid.

Narcotic: Pain-relieving medication that may be addictive.

NCV: See Nerve conduction velocity.

Nerve Conduction Velocity (NCV): Test to determine the speed at which an electrical impulse travels along a nerve.

Nerve Roots: Nerve segments from the spinal cord to where anterior and posterior roots join to form a spinal nerve; Nerves within the vertebral canal and foramina are commonly called roots.

Neurological Surgeon: See Neurosurgeon.

Neurologist: Medical doctor who specializes in the nonsurgical care of disorders of the nervous system.

Neurosurgeon: Medical doctor who specializes in surgical care of disorders of the brain, spinal cord, and nerves. *Also called* Neurological surgeon.

NMR: See Nuclear magnetic resonance.

Nonsteroidal: Not composed of or derived from cortisone; not having the effects of cortisone.

Nuclear Magnetic Resonance (NMR): Technique of producing images by passing radio waves through a subject in a magnetic field.

Nucleus Pulposus: Central portion of an intervertebral disc.

Objective Signs: Abnormalities that can be observed by an examiner without the cooperation of the subject, as opposed to *subjective signs.*

Omentum: Loose folds of supporting tissue around the intestines; commonly a site of fat storage.

Orthopedic: Related to the diagnosis and treatment of disorders of the spine, arms, and legs.

Orthopedic Surgeon: Medical doctor who specializes in diagnosis and treatment, including surgery, of disorders of the spine, arms, and legs. *Also called* Orthopedist.

Orthopedist: See Orthopedic surgeon.

Osteoarthritis: Commonest of the inflammatory joint disorders; also includes wear-and-tear, degenerative joint changes.

Osteopathy: Medical discipline originally based upon spinal manipulation, now evolved to principles similar to those embraced by medical doctors; osteopaths have a D.O. degree from a school of osteopathy.

Osteophyte: Localized enlargement of bone, usually at a site of ligament insertion. *Also called* Bone spur *or* Spur.

Osteoporosis: Weakened state of bones associated with decreased mineral content.

Pain Clinic: Team of specialists working together to provide care for chronic pain problems.

Passive Exercise: Exercise by application of an outside force to the subject; the subject makes no muscular effort.

Pedicle: Side wall portion of a vertebra.

Pelvic Bones: Three bones—the ilium, the ischium, and the pubis—joined to form each side of the pelvis; together they connect the femur to the sacrum.

Pelvic Tilt: Position achieved by rolling the pelvis forward, flattening the lower back, tightening the abdomen, and squeezing the buttocks together.

Pelvis: Lowest portion of the trunk.

Physiatrist: Medical doctor who specializes in rehabilitation from physical deformity and dysfunction.

Physical Impairment: See Impairment.

Physical Therapist: Professional who administers physical treatment measures and guides rehabilitation.

Placebo: Treatment designed to have no direct effect other than psychological.

Plaintiff: Person who brings a lawsuit, such as suing for damages caused by negligence of another.

Polymyalgia Rheumatica: A disease of unknown origin which results in aching pain in trunk muscles, fever, and elevated blood sedimentation rate; often associated with inflammation of the temporal artery.

Polymyositis: A disease which results in generalized inflammation of muscles.

Positive Feedback Cycle: Cycle of events wherein an effect causes a reaction that increases the original effect. *Also called* Vicious cycle or vicious circle (when the effect is detrimental).

Posterior: Toward the back; opposite of *anterior*.

Processes: With reference to bone, outgrowths on the bone that serve as attachment areas for ligaments and tendons.

Prone: Lying face down, back up, on the abdomen.

Prostate: Gland in the male located between the base of the penis and the rectum.

Psoriasis: A form of chronic skin disease, sometimes associated with arthritis.

Psychiatrist: Medical doctor who specializes in the diagnosis and treatment of mental and behavioral disorders.

Psychologist: Nonmedical professional who specializes in the diagnosis and treatment of mental and behavioral disorders.

Psychotherapy: Treatment based upon the discovery of behavior and thought processes and appropriate modifications of them.

Pushoffs: Exercises done prone by pushing the upper body up with the arms while the lower body remains flat.

Quadriceps: Muscles of the front of the thigh.

Radiation: With reference to medical concerns, means ionizing radiation; the effects of x rays.

Radiologist: Medical doctor who specializes in diagnosis through construction of images of the interior of the body, usually by using x rays.

Recertification: Plan that requires periodic medical examination to determine fitness for work, usually to fulfill requirements for a disability benefit.

Rehabilitation Specialist: Professional who works to help with vocational readjustments for handicapped people.

Reiter's Syndrome: Coexistence of particular types of eye infection, inflammation of the urinary tract, and arthritis.

Rest Position: Knees and hips flexed and elevated with the lower back supported.

Restorative: Bringing back to a state of feeling rested and having energy restored.

Rheumatoid Spondylitis: See Ankylosing spondylitis.

Rheumatologist: Medical doctor who specializes in the diagnosis and treatment of arthritis.

Rupture: Breaking out from normal confines; with reference to the intervertebral disc, extrusion of nucleus outside the anulus.

Sacroiliac Joint: Paired joints that connect the sacrum to the pelvis.

Sacrum (Sacral, adjective): Large vertebra at the base of the spine; formed by five vertebrae grown together; connects lumbar spine to pelvis.

Sciatic: Area of the sciatic nerve, the large nerve that forms from nerve roots and courses behind the hip and down the back of the thigh.

Scintimetry: See Bone scan.

Scoliosis: Lateral (side-to-side) curvature of the spine.

Segment: With reference to the spine, two adjacent vertebrae with their adjoining facet joints and disc.

Sedimentation Rate: Test done on blood; values above normal are found in a large variety of disorders, so are not specific to any one disease.

Side Glide: Movement of the upper body directly sideways over the pelvis while the hips stay level.

Side Stretch: Exercise that manipulates the joints of the lower back by putting a direct lateral stretching force upon them.

Side Stretch Roll: Exercise that manipulates the joints of the lower back by putting a lateral stretching force upon them and then adding a twisting force.

Social Security Disability: Benefits provided through government agencies to those who are unable to work because of impairment of health.

Spasm: Muscle tightness that is not under voluntary control.

Spinal Cord: Extension of the brain from the base of the skull to the upper portion of the lumbar spine; connects all spinal nerves to the brain.

Spinal Nerve: Nerve formed by roots from the spinal cord.

Spine: Bony structure of the back; includes 33 bones and the ligaments that bind them.

Spinous Process: Posterior, midline protrusion of bone from each vertebra.

Spondylitis: Inflammation of the spine, either from infection or arthritis.

Spondyloarthropathy: Arthritic disease of the spine.

Spondylolisthesis: Forward displacement of one vertebra relative to an adjacent vertebra.

Spondylolysis: Area in a vertebra composed of fibrous tissue where bone normally exists, usually in the bridge of bone between the facets.

Spondylosis: Condition of the spine characterized by osteophytes and disc degeneration.

Spur: See Osteophyte.

Stenosis: Narrowing of a hollow tube; with reference to the spine, narrowing of the vertebral canal, lateral recess, or intervertebral foramen.

Steroid (Steroidal, adjective): *See* Corticosteroid.

Subcutaneous: Deepest layer of the skin; site for deposit for much of body fat.

Subjective Signs: Manifestations of a disorder that depend upon the information supplied by the subject or upon cooperation of the subject, as opposed to *objective signs.*

Supine: Face up; lying on the back.

Systemic Lupus Erythematosis: A disease of unknown origin which may affect multiple organs.

Tendinitis: Inflammation of tendons, usually where they connect with bone.

Tension: Tightness; loss of the normal ability to relax.

Thermography: Image created by mapping temperature patterns.

Thoracic: Area of the thorax or chest; with reference to the spine, the 12 vertebrae to which ribs are attached.

Tort: Negligent act that results in injury or loss.

Tort System: Part of the legal justice system that deals with torts.

Traction: Pulling or stretching force.

Tranquilizer: Drug used to decrease anxiety, tension, or fear.

Tricyclic Antidepressants: Group of drugs used to relieve depression; also used in the treatment of chronic pain.

Trochanter: Bony knob on a long bone; site of tendon attachments.

Trochanteric Bursa: Bursa sac that lies next to a trochanter; usually refers to the bursa next to the greater trochanter at the side of the hip.

Trochanteric Bursitis: Inflammation of the trochanteric bursa at the hip.

Tumor: Mass or enlarged area; often refers to mass created by abnormal growth of cells, not necessarily cancer.

Ulcerative Colitis: Inflammatory disease of the large bowel sometimes accompanied by arthritis.

Ultrasound: Sound waves used to locate and map internal organs and masses; also used to create deep heat in physical therapy.

Ureter: Tube from the kidney to the bladder.

Valsalva: Effort to increase pressure within the chest and abdomen by making a muscular effort to exhale air against closed nasal and oral airways. *Also called Valsalva Maneuver.*

Valsalva Maneuver: See Valsalva.

Vertebra: Single bony element of the spine.

Vertebral Canal: Tunnel that runs through the spine from the head to the sacrum; spinal cord and spinal nerves pass through it.

Vicious Cycle (or Vicious Circle): See Positive feedback cycle.

Vocational Rehabilitation: Effort to regain fitness to be gainfully employed.

Wall Slides: Exercise done by flattening the back against a wall and bending the knees.

Wolfe's Law: Principle of bone physiology stating that bones get stronger in response to stress.

Yellow Ligament: See Ligamentum flavum.

INDEX